T0091987

Using Occupational Therapy Models in Practice

SECOND EDITION

SECOND EDITION

Using Occupational Therapy Models in Practice

A Fieldguide

MERRILL TURPIN
Senior Lecturer in Occupational Therapy
School of Health and Rehabilitation Sciences
The University of Queensland
QLD 4072 Australia

JENNIFFER GARCIA
Lecturer
School of Occupational Sciences
Universidad del Desarrollo
Santiago, Chile

MICHAEL K. IWAMA
Professor
Department of Orthopedic Surgery
Occupational Therapy Doctorate Division
School of Medicine, Duke University
Durham, USA

ELSEVIER

© 2024, Elsevier Limited. All rights reserved.

No part of this publication may be reproduced or transmitted in any form or by any means, electronic or mechanical, including photocopying, recording, or any information storage and retrieval system, without permission in writing from the publisher. Details on how to seek permission, further information about the Publisher's permissions policies and our arrangements with organizations such as the Copyright Clearance Center and the Copyright Licensing Agency, can be found at our website: www.elsevier.com/permissions

This book and the individual contributions contained in it are protected under copyright by the Publisher (other than as may be noted herein).

Notices

Practitioners and researchers must always rely on their own experience and knowledge in evaluating and using any information, methods, compounds or experiments described herein. Because of rapid advances in the medical sciences, in particular, independent verification of diagnoses and drug dosages should be made. To the fullest extent of the law, no responsibility is assumed by Elsevier, authors, editors or contributors for any injury and/or damage to persons or property as a matter of products liability, negligence or otherwise, or from any use or operation of any methods, products, instructions, or ideas contained in the material herein

ISBN: 978-0-323-87949-1

Content Strategist: Clodagh Holland-Borosh
Content Project Manager: Shivani Pal
Design: Bridget Hoette

Printed in India

Last digit is the print number: 9 8 7 6 5 4 3 2 1

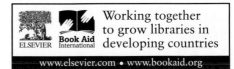

TABLE OF CONTENT

Preface to 2nd Edition   vi

Acknowledgements   ix

Introduction   1

1   Theory and Practice   12

2   Professional Reasoning in Context   22

3   Occupational Performance Models and Occupational Adaptation   39

4   Ecological Models   66

5   Occupational Therapy Practice Framework (OTPF) and Occupational Therapy Intervention Process Model (OTIPM)   87

6   The Model of Human Occupation (MOHO)   113

7   The Canadian Model of Occupational Participation (CanMOP)   136

8   Kawa Model   157

9   Reflections on Occupational Therapy Concepts   173

Index   178

As occupational therapy forges ahead into its second century, the time seemed right to take stock of its current approach to theory and practice. Over the last century, much has changed in this great profession in terms of its ideas and practices. The industrialized world has moved from a period of modernity that favoured singular, positivist explanations of human phenomena and truth, to a post-modern condition marked by plural and relative views of truth and the world around us. The primacy and meanings of 'doing' in contemporary occupational therapy interpreted through the lens of the rational individual is being challenged and expanded to include the possibilities that come with diverse views of truth and collective experience. What was once a biomedically dominated body of theory and knowledge is expanding into the realms of critical social science and social justice. Many of these alterations have been prompted by changes in the greater contexts within which occupational therapy ideas and practices have existed. The evolution of our ideas and theory attest to the enduring occupational therapy belief that humans carry enormous capacity to adapt to diverse environments and their varying circumstances.

As much as these changes present enormous challenges for the occupational therapy scholar and theorist who must find a way to explain the phenomena and shared experiences around 'doing', the challenges for occupational therapy students and practitioners to comprehend and navigate the occupational therapy theory-to-practice continuum across a landscape of diverse contexts of daily life and practice has to be an even more daunting one. Thus, the authors, who have practised and taught occupational therapy theory for almost a century combined, saw the need for a different kind of textbook on occupational therapy models.

When planning the first edition, we felt that what was needed was a textbook that presented a uniform overview of the more popular models of the profession, and one that was written from the perspectives of *practice* and the *practitioner*. We heard and empathized with many practising occupational therapists around the world who were feeling inadequately prepared to use theories and imperatives for practice that were thought up and theorized in locations far removed from the proving grounds of practice. What was really needed in occupational therapy education and practice was a useful resource that students and practitioners could take into and use within varying contexts of the occupational therapy practice arena; one that would help them make the necessary connection between theory and what actually takes place in that crucial dynamic uniting client and therapist. The need to support our colleagues in the field to use theory to help their clients solve the challenges of day to day living led to the infusion of *clinical (professional) reasoning* into the material.

The authors of the first edition recognized a need for a book on occupational therapy theory that would consider the emerging challenge that culture presented to occupational therapy practice in a global world. In the first edition, we stated:

Instead of merely conveying instructions on how a particular model should be applied, a new kind of theory resource that would aim to empower and enable the therapist to critically understand models and how to judiciously select and apply them, was required. With such ideas and tensions in mind, and while the authors contemplated their various needs in occupational therapy theory classes in Australia, North America, the UK and Europe, Asia, South America, and Africa, the basic framework and content of this book you are now examining was born.

Since that edition, awareness has been increasing of the embeddedness of many long-held occupational therapy ideas in a Western/Global North perspective. No longer does the profession assume that models can simply be plucked from their countries of origin and planted without modification in another country. The need for cultural sensitivity, reflexivity and appropriateness is widely acknowledged. The profession has come a long way from the first decade of the twenty-first century when the Kawa model was a lone voice lamenting lack of cultural appropriateness. In contemporary models and editions in this second edition, many Western, traditional taken-for-granted concepts in occupational therapy theory born of individualism, such as independence and client-centredness, have been replaced with relationship-oriented ideas. Structural issues of power intertwined in the client, therapist and institution dynamic, affecting how practitioners reconcile what they want to do, and how they will do it, with their clients are also acknowledged in some models.

This second edition includes a memory aide for each model to assist occupational therapists to use the models in practice, as in the first edition. A new feature of this edition is the inclusion of case illustrations. Because the authors are culturally connected to different countries, we hope that the case studies resonate with occupational therapists in different places in the world.

While not claiming to be a historical document, this book places those theoretical frameworks that aim to guide practice into a broader historical and situational context. Ideas and practices are located in time and space. They exist within a historical context in which they follow on from what has come before and they pave the way for what might come in the future. They also sprout from the fertile soil of other ideas and practices that surround them, both locally and more broadly. As a profession where theory and practice are intimately linked, occupational therapy has a rich tradition of developing conceptual models that aim to guide practice. However, these models of practice also form part of a century-old development of ideas and practices. We believe that no single model is adequate and universally applicable in all occupational therapy situations. Each model is profoundly complex and represents a constellation of conditions, truisms, ideals, cultural norms and values that preceded and now surround them. A similar dance between a model and the contexts of conditions and ideas that contributed to its current form occurs between the model and the unique experiences and circumstances of daily life of the client. The reasoning occupational therapist is the mediator who strives to bring the best and safest fit between the client and what occupational therapy can offer.

This book provides a small window into the progress of theory and practice over the four decades from the 1980s by presenting eleven current occupational therapy models and a review of their historical development. In a rapidly changing world, it is easy to lose sight of what had led up to the current situation and to only look towards the future. However, in doing so, we risk losing important ideas that might have temporarily been put aside in favour of ones that meet current challenges. We hope that this book will assist occupational therapists to review some of the ideas that have been important over the past three decades and to 'dust them off', look at them anew and determine their utility in the current context.

[Merrill] The writing of this book also has its own history. The seeds of the first edition grew out of an invitation from the Division of Occupational Therapy at The University of Queensland to Professor Michael Iwama to become an adjunct professor. His acceptance of this position provided the opportunity for the forging of many important professional relationships for occupational therapy staff members at The University of Queensland. The first edition of this book is the result of one such association (but only one of many). Five years after the first edition was published, Jenniffer Garcia came to Australia from South America to undertake a research higher degree at the Division of Occupational Therapy at The University of Queensland. While my eyes to culture had been opened earlier by Professor Iwama, close collaboration for many years with Dr Garcia has left me with a wide-eyed cultural lens. When it came time for a second edition, it was clear to me that inviting Dr Garcia to be an author would bring even more cultural richness to the text. I wish to thank both Jenniffer and Michael for sharing their wisdom with me, for schooling me in true cultural diversity, and for their passion and breadth of vision for occupational therapy.

[Michael] I remember how blessed and fortunate I felt when I arrived at The University of Queensland in 2003 to begin this wonderful association with the occupational therapists of Australia. I was stunned & impressed by the highly experienced, learned and capable academic team there. I was most impressed in particular by an emerging light in our profession by the name of Merrill Turpin. Though I was initially invited to share ideas about culture and theory in OT with my Australian colleagues, I ended up being schooled by Dr Turpin on these subjects. As you read through this text, you will readily appreciate that the majority of content is Merrill Turpin's. It has been a privilege to 'piggy-back' on Dr Turpin's ideas and work, to be inspired and to be allowed to partner with her in bringing this resource to the classrooms and practice arenas of our great profession. Theory construction, testing, application and evolution are dynamic, fluid processes that necessarily require multiple critical lenses and varying spheres of experience. This edition is strengthened and enriched by co-author Jenniffer Garcia of South America, who broadens even further the critical, cross-cultural lens required to extend justice and inclusion to occupational therapy's diverse, world-wide clientele.

[Jenniffer] For the last eight years I have had the true honour of working with and learning from Dr. Turpin, who has been my mentor, advisor and friend. I graduated as an occupational therapist in Chile 20 years ago, but I moved to Australia because of the lack of disciplinary post-graduate studies in my country. Language barriers, lack of awareness of the resources available, and limited knowledge locally created in the Spanish language, limited the quality of my practice with clients. My journey as MPhil and PhD student at The University of Queensland allowed me to have access to a wide body of knowledge that was not available to me before. I learned about models of practice and theories, frameworks to guide clinical reasoning, and a big range of information that supports research, education and practice of occupational therapists in Anglophone countries. It is a huge privilege for me to be a co-author of this book with Dr. Turpin, who has shared with me her wisdom and deep understanding of the principles of our profession, and the singularities of each model. She has increased my capacity to think critically and be culturally sensitive, we combined our experiences to share examples that could be meaningful and clear for students and occupational therapists in different parts of the world. I am also honoured to work with Professor Iwama, who was a pioneer in publishing a model that emerged from non-western countries. His work is an inspiration for me. I hope this book can be a window to observe the progress of occupational therapy globally, to assist reasoning in practice, which can someday be translated into other languages for colleagues in each corner of the world.

We hope that this book will ultimately be the useful resource to students, practitioners and educators that we envisioned. And if knowledge is indeed power, we would like to see that power, customarily ceded to theoretical side of the continuum, transferred to and vetted in the crucible of occupational therapy practice. We hope that in turn, over time, therapists will once again be regarded as the holders of the essence and potential power of occupational therapy. Occupational therapy models should be interpreted and understood through the lens of practice and in the daily life experiences of our clients. Models should ultimately be evaluated by their usefulness in exacting positive change and benefit to its clients and service recipients. Therefore, we hope that the practising occupational therapist will utilize this book in a different way than they might have with previous theory books. We hope that the student and therapist will bring the book into their places of study and work where it can be handily and conveniently referred to, within the domain of occupational therapy practice.

ACKNOWLEDGEMENTS

We all have families whose love and support have sustained us through the long but enjoyable time of writing the manuscript. I [Merrill] would like to thank my husband Iain Renton for the kindness and compassion that pervades his very being. I would also like to thank him for adding his graphic design skills to the book and drawing some of the figures. I [Michael] would like to thank my wife Sharon for her enduing patience with my obsession for my profession. I [Jenniffer] would like to thank my husband Orlando and my children Catalina and Vicente for being my strength and inspiration every day. We would also like to thank Trinity Hutton, the development editor of the book, for developing and negotiating the proposal for a second edition and for her professionalism and patience.

Merrill Turpin
Jenniffer Garcia
Michael Iwama
Brisbane, Australia; Santiago,
Chile; and Vancouver,
Canada & Durham, USA;
2023

Introduction

CHAPTER CONTENTS

A Historical and Contextual Approach   2

Western Models of Health and Systems Theory   3

Historical Progression in Occupational Therapy Theory   7

Using Models in Practice   9

Overview of the Book   9

References   10

The aspects of things that are most important for use are hidden because of their simplicity and familiarity.

Ludwig Wittgenstein

This book is about the practice of occupational therapy. It is about the process that occupational therapists as professionals use to make decisions about professional action. It is also about the ideas that are (or have been) put together into structured frameworks to guide the practice of occupational therapy. In the quotation at the beginning of this Introduction, Ludwig Wittgenstein alluded to the invisibility that occurs when ideas become so accepted by a community that they are no longer noticed or commented upon. Phenomenologists refer to this situation as the *natural attitude*, whereby people can be unaware of the assumptions that shape their perspectives. People internalize sociocultural understandings, which become taken-for-granted ways of comprehending the world. In the professional realm, developing conceptual frameworks can aid awareness of the many assumptions that are so central to a profession but often go unnoticed.

Occupational therapists have a well-developed practice of using conceptual frameworks to make explicit the ideas that form the basis of their practice. The impetus for this might come partly from the fact that much of occupational therapy practice occurs within the context of ordinary daily life. Because of the ordinariness of everyday life, the occupational therapy knowledge base can appear as "common sense." However, occupational therapy's approach to everyday life is quite particular and definitely not the simple internalization of sociocultural norms. Consequently the profession needs to clarify its unique perspective. In Chapter 1 we discuss how the fact that occupational therapists are sought and accepted in society and are able to provide services that others cannot suggests that occupational therapy perspective and knowledge might better be described as "uncommon sense." Occupational therapy conceptual frameworks, which we will refer to as *models* throughout most of this book, are useful for exploring the profession's unique perspective and uncommon sense.

1

As professionals, occupational therapists wrestle daily with the complexities of facilitating the occupational engagement of clients or populations in their societies. Occupational therapists know it is very difficult (perhaps impossible) to identify generalized principles regarding what helps people do what they need and want to do in their daily lives. They know that individuals, who vary considerably in their nature, abilities, and interests, live their lives in very specific but varied contexts. They also know these contexts are very complex—that they include people, places, materials, and equipment and have cultural, spatial, and temporal dimensions.

Occupational therapists know how people think about and experience themselves depends upon their ability to participate in their specific life contexts. The requirements for participation in daily life are as varied as people themselves and their unique life circumstances. Such requirements might include being able to perform specific tasks for themselves or others, performing tasks by themselves or with others, restraining from action in particular situations, and fulfilling the roles expected by themselves, by others in their "group", and by the broader society in which they live.

In this book we propose that the central concern of occupational therapy is *facilitating context-dependent participation through occupation*. This core concern comprises two concepts: (1) context and (2) participation through occupation. First, occupational therapy has always acknowledged the importance of the contexts in which people live to both their experience and their action. People do specific things in specific places at specific historical and chronological times. Occupational therapy has traditionally used the term *environment* to discuss people's situations, but today the word *context* is increasingly being used. Over time, more specific aspects of the environment that influence performance have been identified, as evidenced by the adjectives used to describe environments, namely *physical, social, societal, institutional, political, cultural, temporal*, and *virtual*.

Second, occupational therapy aims to help people participate through occupation in their local situations and broader societies in ways that are meaningful to them. In common usage, the word *participation* means to take part or share in something. From occupational therapy's perspective, engagement in occupation enables people to take part in their communities in their daily lives. However, due to a combination of circumstances and their own capacities, people might have difficulty taking part in their communities, whether those communities comprise family or other social groups and institutions.

A Historical and Contextual Approach

The decisions people make and the things they do often make sense when accompanied by an understanding of the underlying contexts of their experiences. These experiences have temporal and spatial influences; that is, people live and act in specific places at certain times and in the context of their own biographical and social histories. Professions also exist within specific times and places, each with a history that influences its ideas. How those ideas relate to and resonate with current and future societal conditions may determine the usefulness and viability of the profession.

In this book we present 11 conceptual frameworks, most of which are referred to as *models of practice*. We have chosen these models of practice because they tell a story of the development of ideas in occupational therapy (and therefore occupational therapy practice) over the past 60 or so years. As we discuss in Chapter 1, terminology for conceptual frameworks in occupational therapy is inconsistent, and occupational therapists use a wide range of knowledge from both inside and outside the profession. We do not include conceptual or practice frameworks that occupational therapists might use in specific practice areas to provide detailed guidance about specific assessments and interventions (often referred to as *frames of reference*). Rather, by focusing on occupational therapy models of practice, we aim to discuss how occupational therapy theory and practice is (and has been) conceptualized by a range of different authors in different parts of the world.

We have tried to capture how time and place might have influenced the ideas of particular occupational therapy authors by taking a historical approach to the models we present. Some of these models have been updated through several editions. Others were published at an earlier time and have not been updated. Throughout the book we present the most recent edition of the model and discuss its history and any previous editions. Regardless of when they were first (or last) published, the models in this book have been chosen because they encompass many of the important ideas that have shaped current occupational therapy perspectives. Many of the ideas presented in these conceptual models have become embedded within current occupational therapy philosophy and their influence on practice has been enduring. Presenting a range of models that have been developed in the profession will provide practitioners and theorists with a very condensed view of the ideas that have shaped the profession of occupational therapy. Comparisons among models highlight the various ways that different concepts have been presented in the profession, and a historical perspective shows how the profession's ideas have changed and developed over time. We hope this book will encourage readers to see theory and practice as inextricably linked and to use occupational therapy models quite explicitly in their practice. By comprehending the influence of historical context on theory development, current and future occupational therapists may be compelled to critically consider the relevance and importance of occupational therapy models as they currently exist and contribute to the important processes of updating existing models and innovating new ones.

Western Models of Health and Systems Theory

In this section we discuss some theoretical perspectives that particularly shaped early occupational therapy models. First we discuss four periods in occupational therapy's relatively short history that demonstrate variations in its conceptual attention. Then we widen our lens to the broader context of health and present two approaches that have greatly influenced occupational therapy: the biomedical and biopsychosocial (and systems theory) models of health. Finally, we discuss how occupational therapy historically has concentrated on the participation of *individuals* because of its development as a profession in the Western world—particularly in the health sector, which predominantly promotes an individualistic and mechanistic understanding of health. More recently in occupational therapy, this focus on individuals appears to be changing in line with the broader trends within health toward an increasingly contextualized understanding of health, as well as a greater awareness of the cultural situatedness of much of occupational therapy's conceptual work.

Table I.1 outlines four periods in the history of occupational therapy as identified by Reed (2005) and Kielhofner (2009); while there is close alignment between these two classifications, different terms are used to describe each period. Essentially both classifications commence at a time when the ideas that were to become fundamental to occupational therapy were developed. These were often borrowed from other movements, such as the Moral Treatment movement, which is generally associated with humane treatment and acknowledgment of the importance of routines of work and leisure (Peloquin 1989), and the Arts and Crafts movement, which emphasized the therapeutic, medical, diversional, and recreational use of activity (Levine 1987). That initial period was followed by a period in which occupational therapy was founded on the premise that productive and meaningful human action facilitated good health. The third period in occupational therapy's history was characterized by the dominant mechanistic view of humans provided by the biomedical perspective that was prevalent in health in the middle of the 20th century. The fourth and final period was described by both Reed and Kielhofner as a return to the profession's founding principles pertaining to the value of occupation. Whiteford et al. (2000) emphasized that, in this fourth period, occupational therapy was *returning* to a focus on occupation that had always been present in the profession, rather than developing a new direction. They referred to this reaffirmation as a "renaissance of occupation" (p. 61). These four periods in the profession's history

TABLE I.1 ■ Periods in Occupational Therapy History[a]

Reed (2005)			Kielhofner (2009)		
Time	Period and Influences	Characteristics	Time	Paradigm	Characteristics
1800–1899	Preformative period: Moral Treatment movement, Arts and Crafts movement	Ideas from these movements led to occupational therapy practice in mental health institutions	18th and 19th centuries	Moral Treatment preparadigm	Participation in daily activities contributed to health
1900–1929	Formative period: philosophy of pragmatism	Development of foundational terms and concepts	Beginning of 20th century (1900s)	Paradigm of occupation	Interrelatedness of mind, body, and environment to engagement in occupation
1930–1965	Mechanistic period: philosophy of medicine and scientific (quantitative) method	Many formative concepts "forgotten" and new concepts developed	Late 1940s and 1950s	Mechanistic paradigm	Focus on impairments in internal mechanisms: biomechanical, intrapsychic, and neurological
1966–present	Modern period: return of formative ideas and acceptance of qualitative methods	Development of models of practice, extension of understanding of occupation in daily life	1960s–present	Contemporary paradigm: return to occupation	Return to occupation, focus on factors that influence occupational performance

[a]Based on Reed K. An annotated history of the concepts used in occupational therapy. In: Christiansen CH, Baum CM, Bass-Haugen J, eds. Occupational Therapy: Performance, Participation, and Well-Being. 3rd ed. Slack; 2005:567–626. Kielhofner G. Conceptual Foundations of Occupational Therapy. 4th ed. F.A. Davis; 2009.

demonstrate that occupational therapy has both humanist and biomedical roots and an enduring concern for what people do in their daily lives (i.e., occupation).

Evident in these periods or paradigms in occupational therapy is the influence of trends in the broader context of health. We discuss two models of health that particularly influenced occupational therapy. An important early (post-Enlightenment) trend was toward the *biomedical model of health*. This model gradually became the dominant model of health in Western countries through the rise of medicine from the mid-1800s onward. In discussing this model of health, Taylor and Field (2003) explained that the development of medicine is often described in terms of dramatic breakthroughs. As they stated, "In this 'heroic' view of medicine, the struggle for better health is seen as a 'war' waged by doctors and medical scientists against an impersonal enemy called disease on the battleground of the human body" (p. 21). They listed the main assumptions of the biomedical model of health as follows:

- Health is the absence of biological abnormality.
- Diseases have specific causes.
- The human body is likened to a machine to be restored to health through personalized treatments that arrest or reverse the disease process.
- The health of a society is seen as largely dependent on the state of medical knowledge and the availability of medical resources (pp. 21–22).

Taylor and Field (2003) explained that the dominance of the biomedical model of health was consolidated in the 19th and early 20th centuries through the development of hospitals. The biomedical model is an expert model in which the patient is expected to submit (passively) to investigations of their body (directly through medical examination or indirectly through medical technology such as X-ray and MRI) to locate the cause of their health problem. Once the specific cause has been identified, intervention can be implemented to "fix" the problem.

The mechanistic ideas of the biomedical model are most evident in occupational therapy during the period that both Reed and Kielhofner referred to as *mechanistic* (because it was dominated by the *body-as-machine* metaphor) and in the occupational performance models of the 1960s and 1970s (see Chapter 3). These occupational therapy models emphasized the effect on occupational performance of an individual's impairments, referred to in the models as limitations in *performance components*. However, while the biomedical model focuses on the body, a primary characteristic of occupational therapy has remained a contrasting humanistic concern for people *as people*. An occupational therapy perspective conceptualizes people as holistic beings comprising body, mind, and spirit. This holistic perspective is more aligned with the *biopsychosocial model of health*, the second major health model that has influenced occupational therapy theory.

Western health systems embraced a biopsychosocial model of health in the latter part of the 20th century. Initially George Engel published an article advocating for a model of health that went beyond a normative view of the body and a definition of health as the absence of disease. He called it the biopsychosocial model (Engel 1977). As the name suggests, the model acknowledges that biological, psychological, and social aspects of a person's life influence health. This model of health focuses on well-being (which is more than just the absence of disease) and the subjective experience of health (rather than just the physical manifestations of disease). Over time, the biopsychosocial approach has increasingly dominated health, particularly in health service organizations other than hospitals (where a biomedical model still predominates).

The subjective experience of ill health and disability was a major focus of health research in the early 1980s. Based in medical anthropology and known as the *phenomenology of illness*, this research distinguished between disease and the experience of illness (e.g., see Good and DelVecchio Good 1980; Toombs 1992). It demonstrated that the *experience* of ill health is separate, and often different, from disease. For example, a person might be feeling unwell but, according to diagnostic tests, be free from disease. Conversely, others might be diagnosed with disease despite feeling quite well. The biopsychosocial model emphasized a more holistic understanding of health that included both the physical signs of health and disease as well as the subjective experience of illness.

Coinciding in time with the introduction of the biopsychosocial model of health, systems theory also became influential in shaping an understanding of health (this theory had been introduced earlier into biology; see von Bertalanffy 1950). In systems theory an individual is viewed as both being composed of systems and living within broader systems. Thus individuals are conceptualized as consisting of layers of systems, such as cells, organs, and physiological systems; having broader biological and psychological systems; and existing within external systems such as the sociocultural environment. In this theory people are considered open systems, whereby they receive input from the external environment and are also able to act upon that input (this is in contrast to closed systems, which are not open to the external environment). Engels (1977) explained that, while the biopsychosocial model of health was not based on systems theory, it was consistent with it. In occupational therapy, early and later editions of the Person-Environment-Occupation-Performance (PEOP) and Model of Human Occupation (MOHO) models (see Chapters 4 and 6) explicitly made systems theory their basis.

A common criticism of both the biomedical and biopsychosocial models of health is that they focus on individuals (Gerlach et al. 2017; Verhagen 2017). When these models are applied to health, the emphasis is placed on individual responsibility and the focus on behaviors that individuals should undertake to preserve their health. However, a difficulty with this perspective is that some factors which influence health are beyond an individual's control. For example, the structure and culture of a society shape the health of its members. While individualism is often associated with Western societies, they appear to be changing (albeit slowly), with Indigenous and Eastern ways of thinking and acting becoming more available to the Western world and the collective nature of people's lives becoming more overtly acknowledged. As Trentham et al. (2022) stated, "There is increasing awareness and documentation that health and well-being are tied to sociopolitical forces... [and are] sustained through social structures that create disparities in access to health promoting resources known as social and structural determinants of health" (p. 33). In occupational therapy, historically, the emphasis on the individual-in-context has largely focused on the individual. Currently there are increasing calls to attend to context, not just the immediate environments of individuals but the broader sociopolitical and temporohistorical contexts as well.

The quotation provided by Trenton et al. (2022) refers to social and structural determinants of health. The concept of determinants of health forms the basis for both public health and health promotion approaches targeting populations. As Keleher and MacDougall (2016) identified, a determinants approach to health involves situating health and social problems "in the context of broader social, structural and cultural conditions of our society" (p. 5). A determinant of health is "a factor or characteristic that brings about a change in health, either for the better or for the worse" (Reidpath 2004, p. 9). Determinants of health can be categorized as social, environmental, biological, and genetic and can include a diverse range of factors such as exercise, the quality of the water supply, exposure to the sun, and the conditions in which people work and live. This list shows that improving the health of a population cannot be limited to the health system alone and requires a much broader basis for action. An important concept in a health promotion approach is the concept of social determinants of health. The World Health Organization (2022) listed the following as examples of social determinants of health:

- Income and social protection
- Education
- Unemployment and job insecurity
- Working life conditions
- Food insecurity
- Housing
- Basic amenities and the environment
- Early childhood development

- Social inclusion and nondiscrimination
- Structural conflict
- Access to affordable health services of decent quality

Because the structure of society can advantage or disadvantage different groups and therefore their health (e.g., statistically, the wealthiest are the healthiest), an important concern in understanding and addressing social determinants of health relates to inequality. Examples include the unequal distribution of health, asking why some groups in society are healthier than others, and equity of access to health services. Social determinants also include factors that are protective of health such as safe working conditions.

As we explore in depth in this book more recent versions of the models as well as their histories, we will see a general trend of moving away from a purely individual focus and toward acceptance of a broader concept of "client". This broader concept includes groups and populations and is informed by a determinants approach to population health. This trend is evident in occupational therapy models which attend more explicitly to structural disadvantages facing different groups in society. There is also greater acknowledgment of the Western-centric perspective embedded in many occupational therapy models. With such acknowledgment, some of the more recent models recognize and seek to address collective and more diverse sociocultural perspectives.

Historical Progression in Occupational Therapy Theory

The way that occupational therapy has organized its concepts has changed substantially over time. To facilitate reading this section Table I.2 details the models covered in this book, their various years of publication, and the perspective/model of health underpinning the most recent version. During the 1970s, authors primarily aimed to make explicit the fundamental beliefs of occupational therapy. At that time, these thinking frameworks generally were not called models and were focused on developing a conceptual system that integrated major ideas about interventions for particular population groups. In the late 1970s and continuing during the 1980s, concepts were organized into schemes referred to as *models*. This later phase is characterized by occupational performance models published by the American and Canadian occupational therapy associations. While attending to roles, occupational performance areas (e.g., activities of daily living, work, and leisure), and occupational performance components (e.g., sensory, motor, cognitive, perceptual, psychological, and social), occupational therapy practice was strongly influenced by a biomedical understanding of health and centered on remediation of impairments. A subsequent major criticism of these models was that they were too focused on activities aiming to remediate occupational performance components and were not targeted at the level of occupation. This criticism resonates with contemporary descriptions of models, which frequently contrast an occupational focus with activity-based remediation and a normative view of bodies.

The models first developed in the 1980s generally used the language of systems theory. This represented a first step away from a biomedical understanding and toward the notion of a holistic system. In the 1990s the trend in occupational therapy models might best be described as an entrenchment of the *ecological turn* that had commenced in the 1980s. Person-in-environment was seen as an integrated whole comprising mutually influencing components or parts. For example, many models of this time were particularly influenced by biopsychosocial and systems understandings of humans, explicitly attending to both the components of occupational performance (based on the impairment focus of the biomedical model of health) as well as subjective experiences and psychological concerns such as identity (consistent with a biopsychosocial perspective). The 1990s especially demonstrated a widespread affirmation that occupational therapy was concerned with people's experiences and that these experiences were shaped by their contexts. For example, psychological concepts such as stress were explored because people's health could be influenced by their experiences of their sociocultural environments. In attending to the broader systems surrounding the individual, these occupational therapy models identified different aspects of the

TABLE I.2 ■ Occupational Therapy Models Covered in this Book

Model	Publication Year(s)	Perspective/Model of Health
Occupational Performance Model (OPM) (Pedretti)	1981, 1985, 1990, 1996, 2001	Primarily biomedical
Occupational Performance Model (Australia) (OPM(A)) (Chapparo and Ranka)	1997, 2017	Biopsychosocial
Occupational Adaptation Model (OAM) (Schkade and Schultz)	1992, 1997, 2001, 2003, 2009	Biopsychosocial
Person-Environment-Occupation (PEO) model (Law et al.)	1996	Ecological/biopsychosocial (called transactive because the event is the unit of focus rather than the individual; considers objective and subjective aspects of person)
Ecology of Human Performance (EHP) model (Dunn, Brown, and McGuigan)	1994	Ecological/biopsychosocial (context is the lens through which occupational performance is viewed)
Person-Environment-Occupation-Performance (PEOP) model (Christiansen and Baum)	1991, 1997, 2005, 2015	Ecological/biopsychosocial/systems theory
Occupational Therapy Practice Framework (OTPF-4) (American Occupational Therapy Association [AOTA])	2002, 2008, 2014, 2020	Transactional
Occupational Therapy Intervention Process Model (OTIPM)	1998, 2009, 2019	Transactional
Model of Human Occupation (MOHO) (Kielhofner)	1985, 1995, 2002, 2008	Systems theory
Canadian Model of Occupational Participation	2022 (previous Canadian models 1997, 2002, 2007)	Transactional
Kawa model (Iwama)	2006	Doesn't conform to the major Western models of health (Western practitioners have to be careful that they don't interpret it from a biopsychosocial perspective)

environment with which the individual interacted. For example, in contrast to earlier occupational performance models that acknowledged context generically, occupational therapy models in this decade emphasized the specific *contexts* in which people lived. This prompted a consequent increased attention to the environment, detailing a variety of environmental characteristics such as physical, sensory, social, institutional, economic, and cultural. Another feature of this ecological turn was expansion from the individualist notion of occupational performance to include broader concepts such as participation and engagement in society.

Two models published during the 1990s, Ecology of Human Performance (EHP, Dunn 1994) and Person-Environment-Occupation (PEO, Law et al. 1996), stand out as presenting the relationship among people, their context, and what they are doing as an intertwined whole. Both models drew upon the ecological notions emphasized in science at the time and presented people as richly embedded with contexts that shape them and what they do, as well as being shaped by them and their action. We especially highlight these two models because they predate the emphasis on a transactional perspective that has recently become more widely adopted.

While the 1990s was a period marked by substantial model development and refinement, only one occupational therapy model was developed in the subsequent decade. The Kawa model

(Iwama 2006) specifically addressed the cultural assumptions underpinning occupational therapy, highlighting and providing an alternative to the profession's taken-for-granted Western perspective. In the intervening time since that model was published, much discussion of concepts such as cultural awareness, cultural relevance, cultural sensitivity, and cultural safety has ensued. For example, discussions often demonstrate increased awareness and critique of the cultural bias inherent in many occupational therapy concepts such as independence and the categorization of occupation into self-care, work, and leisure.

We describe the major direction evident in changes to many contemporary models as a *transactional turn*. Whereas the models of the 1990s took an ecological turn and emphasized that it is the person in context that performs or participates in occupation, the transactional turn takes situatedness to a whole new level. The concept of people as separate entities is no longer at the center of contemporary models, as it was in client-centered practice, and instead has largely disappeared from these models. Whereas occupation was previously imagined as something done by people, it has been more recently understood as the *result* of the transaction of many factors (only one of which is the person). Occupation is situated within transactional relationships among time, place, culture, relationships, people, animals, history, and social structures. While the Kawa model was developed in the first decade of this century and particularly focused on cultural issues, it could be seen to share a transactional perspective. Rather than being person centered, it presents a decentralized self that is one with all that surrounds it, with life flowing through this integrated whole. It does not share Western values and has a unique cultural perspective.

Using Models in Practice

This book is about using models in practice rather than just understanding them as an end in themselves. Models essentially provide an organizing framework for thinking about practice in a systematic way and a language with which to discuss practice with others. Professional practice is recognized as a complex and messy process. Without some process for making sense of the complicated situations in which therapists find themselves, professional practice can become haphazard and dependent upon individual occupational therapists.

Models of practice in occupational therapy articulate the beliefs and values of the profession. They develop from practice concerns and provide frameworks for systematically addressing them. As Kielhofner (2009) stated, "a model is only useful if it is thoroughly grounded in practice" (p. 62). Models of practice provide a language to help individual occupational therapists articulate to others the perspective that is unique to their profession. They make explicit the concepts upon which the profession is based and how concepts are grouped or organized. Thus they are important for strengthening the professional identities of occupational therapists by providing a language with which to express to others their habitual ways of making sense of the world and the value of their professional perspective for their clients.

Trede and Higgs (2008) stated that "models can be thought of as mental maps that assist practitioners to understand their practice" (p. 32). This is the way we conceptualize them in this book. By exploring the different models of practice in detail in this one text, we hope to provide readers with a resource that helps them compare and contrast the different occupational therapy models and select models that support the professional reasoning they need to do in certain contexts at specific historical times. We also hope this condensed presentation of occupational therapy models of practice helps readers distill the essence of occupational therapy philosophy.

Overview of the Book

To facilitate the use of models in practice, this book aims to provide an overview of a range of different occupational therapy models, placed within the conceptual context of practice. As a field guide it aims to provide a resource for occupational therapists and occupational therapy students while engaged in professional practice. Chapters 1 and 2 provide a context within which to think about the use of models in practice. Chapter 1 discusses the concepts of theory and practice and how they are related to each other. It presents theory as a way of thinking that arises from and aims to make sense of practice. It also discusses the different types and sources of knowledge that occupational therapists might use in practice. Chapter 2 explores the nature of professional practice and uses the concept of professional reasoning to explore how models can be used to guide what occupational therapists "see" in their practice and how they think about it, which, in turn, guides what they do. It presents the Model of Context-specific Professional Reasoning (MCPR), which outlines the perspectives that occupational therapists and the people with whom they work bring to a professional encounter, the various layers of context that shape their work, and the unique reasoning-in-action process they undertake. This chapter includes a case to illustrate use of the MCPR. Chapters 3 through 8 provide an overview of 11 occupational therapy models. These chapters begin with a description of the model's purpose, structure, and concepts, along with a diagrammatic representation of the model. Following this, the historical development of the model is discussed. To facilitate the model's use in practice, a memory aid is provided to guide clinicians when using the model. The major works relating to each model are also provided. To help readers see some of the similarities in the various models, some are grouped within one chapter. For example, Chapter 3 focuses on individual occupational performance and adaptation and includes one occupational performance model from the United States and one from Australia, as well as the Occupational Adaptation model. Chapter 4 includes three models that all take an ecological approach to person and occupation in environment. Chapter 5 provides an overview of the following two contemporary models from the United States: the fourth edition of the Occupational Therapy Practice Framework: Domain and Process (OTPF-4) and the Occupational Therapy Intervention Process Model (OTIPM). A case is also provided to illustrate use of these two models in practice. Then, three models are presented in separate chapters as their organization and/or emphasis differs from some of the other models. These three chapters also include case illustrations. Chapter 6 discusses the Model of Human Occupation (MOHO), Chapter 7 presents the Canadian Model of Occupational Participation, along with the Collaborative Relationship-Focused Occupational Therapy approach and the Canadian Occupational Therapy Inter-Relational Practice Process Framework. And Chapter 8 reviews the Kawa model, with its emphasis on a decentralized self within a collectivist culture. Finally, Chapter 9 provides a conclusion to the book.

References

Dunn W, Brown C, McGuigan A. The ecology of human performance: a framework for considering the effect of context. *Am J Occup Ther.* 1994 Jul;48(7):595–607. doi:10.5014/ajot.48.7.595

Engel GL. The need for a new medical model: a challenge for biomedicine. *Science.* 1977 Apr 8;196(4286): 129–136. doi:10.1126/science.847460

Gerlach AJ, Teachman J, Laliberte-Rudman D, Aldrich R, Huot S. Expanding beyond individualism: engaging critical perspectives on occupation. *Scand J Occup Ther.* 2018;25(1):35–43. doi:10.1080/11038128.20 17.1327616

Good B, DelVecchio Good MJ. The meaning of symptoms: a cultural hermeneutic model for clinical practice. In: Eisenberg I, Kleinman A, eds. *The Relevance of Social Science for Medicine.* Reidel; 1980:165–196.

Iwama M. *The Kawa Model: Culturally Relevant Occupational Therapy.* Churchill Livingstone; 2006.

Keleher H, MacDougall C, eds. Concepts of health. In: *Understanding Health.* Oxford University Press; 2016:3–18.

Kielhofner G. *Conceptual Foundations of Occupational Therapy.* 4th ed. F.A. Davis; 2009.

Law M, Cooper B, Strong S, Stewart D, Rigby P, Letts L. The Person-Environment-Occupation model: a transactive approach to occupational performance. *Can J Occup Ther.* 1996 Apr;63(1):9–23. doi:10.1177/000841749606300103

Levine RE. The influence of the arts-and-crafts movement on the professional status of occupational therapy. *Am J Occup Ther.* 1987 Apr;41(4):248–254. doi:10.5014/ajot.41.4.248

Peloquin SM. Moral treatment: contexts considered. *Am J Occup Ther.* 1989 Aug;43(8):537–544. doi:10.5014/ajot.43.8.537

Reed K. An annotated history of the concepts used in occupational therapy. In: Christiansen CH, Baum CM, Bass-Haugen J, eds. *Occupational Therapy: Performance, Participation, and Well-Being.* 3rd ed. Slack; 2005:567–626.

Reidpath D. Social determinants of health. In: Keleher H, Murphy B, eds. *Understanding Health: A Determinants Approach.* Oxford University Press; 2004:9–22.

Taylor S, Field D. Approaches to health and health care. In: Taylor S, Field D, eds. *Sociology of Health and Health Care.* Blackwell; 2003:21–42.

Toombs SK. *The Meaning of Illness: A Phenomenological Account of the Different Perspectives of Physicians and Patient.* Kluwer Academic Publishers; 1992.

Trede F, Higgs J. Collaborative decision making. In: Higgs J, Jones M, Loftus S, Christensen N, eds. *Clinical Reasoning in the Health Professions.* 3rd ed. Butterworth Heinemann; 2008:31–41.

Trentham B, Laliberte-Rudman D, Smith H, Phenic A. The socio-political and historical context of occupational therapy in Canada. In: Egan M, Restall G, eds. *Promoting Occupational Participation: Collaborative Relationship-Focused Occupational Therapy.* Canadian Association of Occupational Therapists; 2022:31–35.

Verhagen PJ. Psychiatry and religion: consensus reached! *Mental Health, Religion & Culture.* 2017;20(6):516–527. doi:10.1080/13674676.2017.1334195

Von Bertalanffy L. The theory of open systems and biology. *Science.* 1950 Jan 13;111(2872):23–29. doi:10.1126/science.111.2872.23

Whiteford G, Townsend E, Hocking C. Reflections on a renaissance of occupation. *Can J Occup Ther.* 2000 Feb;67(1):61–69. doi:10.1177/000841740006700109

World Health Organization. Social Determinants of health. Accessed 25/10/2022. https://www.who.int/health-topics/social-determinants-of-health#tab=tab_1

CHAPTER 1

Theory and Practice

CHAPTER CONTENTS

What Are Theory and Practice and
Why Do They Matter?   12

Practice Is More Than Theory   13

Different Types of Knowledge   13

Implications of Different Types
of Knowledge   15

Terminology   15

Practice as a Starting Point: Models Serving
Occupational Therapy Practice   18

How Models of Practice Serve Practice   19

Conclusion   20

References   21

In this book, and beginning with this chapter, we draw upon the idea that different ways of knowing are required for practice. Rather than taking the perspective that theory precedes and is applied to practice, we use practice as our starting point and ask how theory can *serve* practice.

What Are Theory and Practice and Why Do They Matter?

Theory is a system of connected ideas or concepts intended to explain a phenomenon. It can be used to guide or inform action. As Cohn and Coster (2019) explained, "theories help practitioners reason about what to assess, how to understand occupational performance problems, how to intervene, and what to expect from intervention" (pp. 584–585). They help practitioners articulate their reasoning to others by providing a framework for making reasoning explicit. When theories are made explicit they can be scrutinized and tested.

Practice involves delivering a service and requires reasoned action. In occupational therapy, the terms *clinical reasoning*, *professional reasoning*, and *occupational reasoning* (Chaparro and Ranka 2019) have been used to label the thinking that underpins decisions about action. In this book we use the term *professional reasoning*. Both reasoning and action are required for practice. Chaparro and Ranka (2019) discussed a range of internal and external influences on occupational therapists' decisions about action. These include the therapy context, clients and their life contexts, theory and professional knowledge, occupational therapists' professional identities, and attitudes to and expectations about service provision.

In this chapter we will see that theory is an essential part of practice, but that simply knowing information is insufficient for practice. While theories form part of a profession's body of knowledge, experienced occupational therapists often have difficulty explaining the theoretical bases for their practice. However, it has long been acknowledged that they make well-reasoned and effective decisions after gaining very little information (Mattingly and Fleming 1994), which suggests that they are skillfully combining the information they obtain in practice with their body of knowledge. They make rapid but well-informed decisions about their practice.

Practice Is More Than Theory

Often, theories are conceptualized as being "applied" to practice, the implication being that theory somehow precedes (and is possibly superior to) practice. Mattingly and Fleming (1994) explained that, in the health professions, the reasoning required has generally been conceptualized as "applied natural science" in which "reasoning is presumed to involve recognizing particular instances of behavior in terms of general laws that regulate the relationship between cause and a resultant state of affairs" and that "practice is considered the application of empirically tested abstract knowledge (theories) and generalizable factual knowledge" (p. 317). Certainly, most occupational therapy programs in Western countries are structured with theoretical concepts taught earlier and more extensive professional practice experiences occurring later. An extensive knowledge of theory is also consistent with society's expectation of professionals as experts. Theory is often associated with knowing and thinking.

While theory appears to be essential for practice, it is rarely considered to be sufficient for it. The practice of occupational therapy refers to what occupational therapists do in their professional roles; that is, the actions they take. In practice, thinking and action are not separate processes, but are intertwined. Often, it is assumed that thinking precedes action, that people plan their action and then implement that plan through action. However, Mattingly and Fleming (2019) explained that "some philosophers, particularly phenomenologists, claim that thought and action occur in a rapid dynamic in relation to one another, not in a fixed sequence" (p. 120). Practice uses a process that requires decision-making about action and can be thought of as reasoned action. In Chapter 2, we present the Model of Context-specific Professional Reasoning (MCPR). This model includes the reasoning-in-action process used by occupational therapists in practice and emphasizes that thinking and action are intertwined processes.

While both theory and practice are important for the work of professionals, they are not the same. In explaining the difference, Turpin and Hanson (2023) referred to Ryle's (1949) distinction between knowing *that* and knowing *how*. Theory can be thought of as knowing *that*. By making explicit what a particular profession knows, theory is essential to both the organization and sharing of the profession's knowledge base in its area of concern. On the other hand, practice is more aligned with knowing *how*. It requires both the skills required for particular aspects of the profession's work and the ability to choose action (or nonaction) wisely. We now turn to examining two different ways of knowing that are associated with knowing *that* and knowing *how*.

Different Types of Knowledge

In discussing the difference between theory and practice, authors often refer to the ancient philosophies of Plato and Aristotle. While both philosophers agreed that there are different types of knowledge, Plato argued for the superiority of the type of knowledge associated with mathematics. This kind of knowledge was called *episteme* and gives rise to the term *epistemology*. This type of knowledge is (1) propositional, in that it comprises a set of assertions or propositions that can be explained, studied, and transmitted in words and often includes assertions of truth; (2) generalized, in that it aims to state universal principles; and (3) purely intellectual (rather than emotional). It is generally associated with a scientific way of thinking and is the type of knowledge that the word *theory* usually conjures.

In contrast, the type of knowledge often associated with practice is *phronesis* or practical wisdom. As Kessels and Korthagen (1996) explained, "this is an essentially different type of knowledge, not concerned with scientific theories, but with the understanding of specific concrete cases and complex or ambiguous situations" (p. 19). This type of knowledge is situated in and relevant to particular times and places. As Aristotle stated in *The Nicomachean Ethics*, while phronesis can involve general principles, "it must take into account particular facts as well, since it is concerned with practical activities, which always deal with particular things" (Aristotle 1975, p. 1141). Understanding a particular situation depends on experience. As practitioners gain experience, they are able to see patterns and similarities in a series of particular instances. As Kessels and Korthagen (1996) explained, "particulars only become familiar with experience, with a long process of perceiving, assessing situations, judging, choosing courses of action, and being confronted with their consequences" (p. 20). As practice experience increases, knowing and action become more difficult to disentangle. Through pattern recognition, experienced practitioners size up situations quickly and respond with action. Similarly, the action and its outcomes increase practitioners' knowledge and understanding of the situation.

In reflecting on these two types of knowledge, we can see that they align very well with the ideas of theory and practice and knowing *that* and *how*. Theory and knowing *that* are the type of knowledge known as *propositional knowledge*, which aligns most closely with the concept of episteme, and is often associated with professions. It is also known as *scientific knowledge* and *declarative knowledge*. Cohn and Coster (2019) defined propositions used in propositional knowledge as "formal statements about causes and effects or the nature of relationships among features of the world" (p. 585). As Turpin and Hanson (2023) explained that propositions are generally stated as facts, such as "the knee is a hinge joint," "fight and flight are common stress responses," and "blue eye color is linked to a recessive gene," and as principles, such as "adolescence is an important stage in identity formation." Facts and principles are often combined into theories such as Developmental Theory and Sociological Theory (Turpin and Hanson 2023). Propositional knowledge is the type of knowledge that underpins the concept of the expert. It forms an important part of the professional knowledge base, which is often associated with broad principles that can be generalized to a range of different settings. Because propositional knowledge can easily be put into words, it can be a vehicle for professions to express their uniqueness and share it publicly.

The type of knowledge that aligns with practice, knowing *how*, and phronesis is *nonpropositional knowledge*, also called *procedural knowledge*. Whereas propositional knowledge is generalized and aims for universal application, nonpropositional knowledge is specific and embodied. It is linked to action rather than pure thought. It is based on experience in practice and relates to knowing how to do something. It includes the skills required to practice; knowing from experience the types of problems that particular client groups might face and the kinds of interventions that are often useful to them; and knowledge about the particular client with whom the professional is working at the time. It is also embodied rather than based on thought or language. For example, when very experienced occupational therapists are asked how to make a splint for a particular client, it is often easier for them to demonstrate or use strategies such as hand over hand, in which the experienced therapist places their hand on the learner and guides their actions, than to verbally explain the process. As an embodied way of knowing, nonpropositional knowledge incorporates personal knowledge, or knowledge of oneself. This includes awareness of one's own personality, interests, preferences, and skills and challenges. It is built up over the course of people's lives and can relate to the social mores they have experienced and internalized or rejected, their world views, and any knowledge of themselves as people that they have developed through reflection and experience.

Another distinction that has been made is between formal and personal theories (Cohn and Coster 2019). Formal theories are those that are publicly articulated and published and are represented by the models of practice in this book. Personal theories are beliefs held by individuals. They are developed through people's experiences and perspectives when observing, participating in, and being exposed to ideas and beliefs. They are not made widely available and therefore are less likely to have been publicly scrutinized and debated.

Implications of Different Types of Knowledge

The distinction between personal and formal theories is important to consider in relation to the current emphasis in health on evidence-based practice (EBP). The desire to provide quality and cost-effective services that have a positive impact on outcomes for clients and patients is widely shared by a range of stakeholder groups including clients, health professionals, managers of services, and funding bodies (Turpin and Higgs 2010). However, there is a lack of consensus as to how to achieve these outcomes. In its approach to achieving these outcomes, the EBP movement generally values formal theories over personal theories. It promotes the use of knowledge that has been generated and tested using rigorous research methods such as randomized controlled trials and their systematic reviews. The emphasis on research findings that are generalizable to situations other than those in which the results were generated aims to overcome the limitations in reasoning that have been noted in professionals. As Duncan (2020) explained, "it is known that professionals' individual perspectives are highly vulnerable to a range of biases and heuristics when making clinical judgements" (p. 38).

A problem facing practitioners is that, if they only rely on their own experiences of phenomena in the local context, they are likely to make their decisions based on a reasonably narrow range of choices. These are often influenced by factors other than effectiveness of interventions. An example includes the difference between a practitioner's extensive knowledge of the services they can provide and their relative lack of knowledge of the interventions another professional or service could provide (and the research outlining the effectiveness or otherwise of these interventions).

On the other hand, the advantage of personal theories is that they are based on experience within a particular practice context and involve the knowledge of and capacity to respond to individual variations in client preferences and needs. In a much-cited definition, Sackett (2000) defined evidence-based medicine (upon which EBP in occupational therapy is based) as "the integration of best research evidence with clinical expertise and patient values" (p. 1). This definition outlines that the process of EBP requires the integration of different types of knowledge and suggests that both formal and personal theories may be constitutive of EBP.

There is much discussion about theory and practice in professional disciplines. In these discussions, frequent reference is made to a "gap" between theory and practice. The concept of the theory–practice gap provides a way of articulating the problem inherent within professional practice of having to integrate different types of knowledge from different sources when making decisions about professional action. While definitions of EBP, such as the one by Sackett (2000) quoted earlier, refer to the integration of different types of information, little has been done to investigate the process of integration.

Valuing and therefore having to combine different types of knowledge in practice is particularly powerful within occupational therapy. The equal valuing of both propositional and nonpropositional knowledge has been expressed in occupational therapy through concepts such as *art and science* and the *two-body practice* (Mattingly and Fleming 1994). In addition, through its focus on occupation as both a means to facilitate occupational performance and participation and an end in itself, the practice of occupational therapy requires both theory about occupation and practical guidance on how to use occupation to achieve these aims (i.e., theory and practice, knowing *that* and *how*, and episteme and phronesis).

Terminology

In this section, a range of different terminology is reviewed in relation to the occupational therapy discourse about theory and practice. A historical approach to understanding this terminology has been taken because the way occupational therapy has referred to theory and practice appears to have changed over time. The various ways that authors have categorized theory are also discussed.

There are historical differences in the way terms have been used to describe the various levels of theory referred to in occupational therapy. Mosey, an important writer about occupational therapy theory in the 1970s, 1980s, and early 1990s, distinguished between a profession's "fundamental body of knowledge" (1992, p. 49) and its "applied body of knowledge" (p. 69). She stated that "a profession's fundamental body of knowledge is a compilation of all the information a profession recognizes as basic to, and supportive of, its applied body of knowledge and practice. The information is typically a combination of philosophical and scientific knowledge drawn from a variety of sources. It may also include some practical knowledge" (p. 49). Mosey identified five categories of knowledge within a profession's fundamental body of knowledge: (1) philosophical assumptions (basic beliefs), (2) an ethical code, (3) theoretical foundations ("theories and empirical data that serve as a scientific basis for practice" [p. 63]), (4) a domain of concern, and (5) legitimate tools.

Mosey (1992) explained that a profession also requires an applied body of knowledge, which is compatible with the fundamental body of knowledge because the latter "is not meant to be used directly" (p. 69). She defined an applied body of knowledge as "a collection of information formulated so that it serves as the basis for day-to-day problem identification and resolution with clients" and proposed that it included a profession's "sets of guidelines for practice" (p. 69). She commented that, while a range of different terms might be used for these guidelines, including terms like *practice theory*, *model of practice*, and *ground rules*, all of these terms refer to "the transformation of theoretical knowledge into a form that allow[s] it to be used in practice" (p. 73).

Mosey (1992) provided examples of two sets of guidelines for practice: (1) diagnostic categories in medicine and (2) frames of reference in occupational therapy. She explained that a frame of reference includes (1) its theoretical base that "defines and describes the nature of the area of human experience to which the frame of reference is addressed" (p. 85); (2) the relevant function–dysfunction continua which define the way problem areas are understood and how they are resolved; (3) the behaviors and physical signs that indicate function and dysfunction; and (4) the postulates (statements or precepts) outlining the actions that are expected to lead to change (usually to enhance function in whatever way it is conceptualized in the frame of reference).

Mosey (1992) conceptualized frames of reference as relevant to a particular profession. For example, she stated, "it should be remembered that a frame of reference is only one type of *sets of guidelines* for practice. Frames of reference are not suitable for medicine, just as diagnostic categories are not suitable for occupational therapy. Each profession, then, has a type of *sets of guidelines* to meet its own particular practice needs" (p. 87).

In contrast to Mosey's definition, subsequent authors often used the term *frame of reference* to refer to bodies of knowledge that occupational therapists use which are *not* specific to occupational therapy. Crepeau et al. (2009) stated that "frames of reference guide practice by delineating the beliefs, assumptions, definitions, and concepts within a specific area of practice". An example of this categorization includes theoretical frameworks such as developmental, cognitive behavioral, psychodynamic, and biomechanical (Reel and Feaver 2006). Categorizing frames of reference as those approaches that guide practice in a specific area means specific perspectives can be included regardless of whether they are specific to occupational therapy or not. Consequently, the examples of frames of reference provided by a number of authors include approaches that are broader than occupational therapy, such as motor control, self-advocacy, and rehabilitation, as well as frameworks that are specific to occupational therapy practice, such as many occupational therapy association practice guidelines.

Writing to a broader interdisciplinary audience, Reel and Feaver (2006) listed eight terms often used to discuss theory and practice in rehabilitation: (1) frames of reference, (2) domains, (3) treatment approaches, (4) paradigms, (5) perspectives, (6) models, (7) philosophies, and (8) techniques. In organizing this list, they first considered philosophy to be a broader concept and cited Craig's 1983 definition as follows: "A philosophy is a creed, a set of beliefs to live by; it provides a purpose encompassing and overriding the minor and trivial concerns of the everyday, or if not, it communicates a state of mind from within which the ultimate purposelessness of life becomes bearable" (p. 53). They proposed that the various disciplines working in rehabilitation have their own philosophies but also have shared philosophies. Examples of the latter are health-care ethics, client-centered practice, and a developmental/lifelong context. They defined professional philosophy as "the system of beliefs and values unique to each profession, which provides its members with a sense of identity and exerts control over theory and practice. It helps locate the domains of concern for that profession — irrespective of the particular practice context" (p. 53). They defined frames of reference as "clusters of theories selected or developed by different professionals out of the need to support the philosophical beliefs that are the core of the profession" and stated that "Frames of reference give principles on which to base specific intervention. Frames of reference are aimed at specific problems and professionals choose from a number of appropriate frames of reference." (p. 55.) In comparing philosophy and frames of reference, they suggested that philosophies (and paradigms) represented a "softer" type of knowledge and that frames of reference are based on the "harder" sciences (p. 56).

The way terms are used in occupational therapy varies widely and is dependent on the system each author uses for classifying different levels of theory. Generally, the term *frame of reference* is favored for theoretical systems that are not specifically limited to the profession of occupational therapy. This term often appears to be used interchangeably with terms such as *treatment* and *intervention approaches* because they often provide a level of detail that enables their direct use in practice. In contrast, theoretical frameworks that deal with occupation are specific to the profession of occupational therapy and these are generally referred to as *conceptual models of practice.*

In occupational therapy, Cole and Tufano (2008) identified three levels of theory: (1) paradigm, (2) occupation-based models, and (3) frames of reference. They used the term *paradigm* to "incorporate some of what Mosey called our fundamental body of knowledge" (p. 57), and included the philosophical basis for occupational therapy, its values and ethics, and "three concepts most basic to practice in the OT profession: occupation, purposeful activity, and function" (p. 57). They drew upon the American Occupational Therapy Association's (AOTA) Occupational Therapy Practice Framework (OTPF), proposing that it creates a classification system "for OT knowledge that is consistent with our paradigm" (p. 59). Cole and Tufano's second level was occupation-based models. They explained that these have also been referred to as *overarching frames of reference, conceptual models*, and *occupation-based frameworks*. They stated that, "in OT, occupation-based models help explain the relationships among the person, the environment, and occupational performance, forming the foundation for the profession's focus on occupation" (p. 57). The following models are included in this level: Occupational Behaviour, Model of Human Occupation, Occupational Adaptation, Ecology of Human Performance, and Person Environment Occupation Performance. Their third level, called *frames of reference*, referred to practice guidelines in specific domains. This level included applied behavioral, cognitive behavioral, biomechanical and rehabilitative, Allen's Cognitive Levels, and a range of other frames of reference.

Kielhofner (2009) presented knowledge relevant to occupational therapy as three concentric circles, with paradigm in the innermost circle, conceptual practice models in the next outer circle, and related knowledge in the outermost circle. *Paradigm* refers to the shared or common vision of the discipline and includes core constructs, a focal viewpoint, and values. Kielhofner proposed that the paradigm helps unify the profession and define its nature and purpose. Conceptual practice models provide the details that guide occupational therapists in their practice, and he contended that they consist of theory, practice resources, and a research and evidence base. In contrast to the previous two layers, related knowledge comprises knowledge and skills that are not unique to occupational therapy. Kielhofner provided examples such as knowledge of medical diagnoses and disease processes, and cognitive and behavioral concepts and skills from psychology.

Duncan's (2020) categorization of levels of theory is consistent with that of Kielhofner (2009). He used three theoretical categories to structure his presentation of occupational therapy frameworks: (1) paradigm, which was defined as "the shared consensus regarding the most fundamental beliefs of the profession" (p. 40); (2) frame of reference, which he conceptualized as a theoretical framework that was developed outside the profession but could be judiciously used in occupational therapy (similar to Kielhofner's related knowledge); and (3) conceptual models of practice, which are occupation focused and developed specifically to explain occupational therapy practice and processes. Examples of conceptual models of practice provided were the Model of Human Occupation (MOHO), the Canadian Model of Occupational Performance and Engagement (CMOP-E), the Person-Environment-Occupation-Performance (PEOP) model, the Occupational Therapy Intervention Process Model (OTIPM), and the Kawa model. The frames of reference provided were the client-centered, cognitive behavioral, and biomechanical frames of reference, as well as the theoretical approaches to movement and cognitive-perceptual dysfunction.

Throughout this book, we have followed the categorization used by Duncan and Kielhofner and have included formal theoretical frameworks called *models of practice* (often abbreviated to *models*). The two exceptions to this inclusion are the Theory of Occupational Adaption and the Occupational Therapy Practice Framework (OTPF). We have not included theoretical or philosophical frameworks, nor specific frames of reference that exist to guide practice in a specific area.

Practice as a Starting Point: Models Serving Occupational Therapy Practice

In this book, we draw on the idea that different ways of knowing are required for practice. Rather than taking the perspective that theory precedes and is applied to practice, we use practice as our starting point and ask how theory can *serve* practice. Emphasizing the difference between "serving" and "applying to" allows us to address the taken-for-granted assumption in Western society that theoretical knowledge has a higher intrinsic value than practical wisdom. We challenge this view that theory either precedes or is of greater value than practice. Instead, we center our attention firmly on how theory can be used in and be a resource for practice. As far back as 1995, Kielhofner stated that "Theory can never tell therapists, in advance, exactly what should be done in the context of therapy. But, if therapists understand a theory, it will help them figure out what to do at the time. Practice requires therapists to imagine how persons might find their ways out of states of dysfunction and achieve better lives. Theory which supports such therapeutic imagining cannot offer a simple plan or recipe. Rather, it must sharpen and deepen the quality of a therapist's thinking." (p. 1.)

Occupational therapy is a practice in which the development of models of practice has been important. We present two ways in which the closely linked nature of theory and practice in occupational therapy may have contributed to the proliferation of models of practice. First, occupational therapy focuses on occupation in everyday life; that is, the "doing" of everyday life. Engagement in occupation and participation in society are generally taken for granted and therefore often invisible until disrupted. Because of the inherent invisibility of ordinary doing, from outside the profession the practice of occupational therapy can appear like "common sense." However, occupational therapy practice could better be described as *uncommon sense* because occupational therapists provide unique ways of looking at various aspects of ordinary doing. They use this unique perspective to enable people in a variety of circumstances to participate fully in their daily lives and societies. However, this uncommon sense and unique perspective needs to be articulated clearly to others who might not notice or understand it. Making it explicit can assist others to see the value of occupational therapy's contribution to people's lives and understand that it is much more than common sense. Without such explicitness, the value of occupational therapy could go unnoticed. Occupational therapy models of practice provide a vehicle for making the profession's uniqueness overt and explicit.

The second reason why models of practice in occupational therapy could have become prolific lies in the profession's basis in pragmatism, a discipline of philosophy. Pragmatism emphasizes the close connection between thought and action (theory and practice). A person's perspective shapes what they choose to do (they act in ways they think are best in specific situations), and it is through action that people acquire knowledge (Madsen and Josephsson 2017). This perspective of pragmatism appears to operate at two levels within occupational therapy. First, occupational therapists are concerned with both what people do and how they think about those actions. This concern is usually articulated through the concept of meaningful and purposeful occupation. That is, people's actions are always meaningful to them (while these meanings are shaped by the social circumstances in which they live, they are unique to each individual) and they serve a purpose in their lives. The second way the connection between thought and action is evident in occupational therapy is in the way occupational therapists work. Mattingly and Fleming (1994) emphasized that occupational therapists reason through action. This is consistent with the perspective of pragmatism that people acquire knowledge through action. Thus the distinction that is often made between theory and practice does not fit well with the way occupational therapists work. While it is accepted that they need to have a firm base of knowledge upon which to ground their practice, occupational therapists quickly turn their knowledge into action, whether it is preexisting generalized knowledge or specific knowledge about clients and their circumstances, and they also acquire new knowledge through action. Models of practice aim to assist therapists by providing a conceptual framework for thinking about, planning, and interpreting action, both their own action and that of their clients. While other levels of theory might aim to address issues such as philosophy, models of practice aim to link theory to practice.

How Models of Practice Serve Practice

Models of practice aim to guide practice by providing a basis for reasoning and decision-making. They are specific to occupational therapy and encapsulate the values and beliefs of the profession. Because occupation is the core of occupational therapy, they all deal with occupation in a central way. Models of practice *serve* practice in a variety of ways.

First, models of practice make the profession's assumptions about humans and occupation explicit. In explaining the relevant concepts and their relationships, each model makes explicit the assumptions upon which it is based. For the model to be accepted as appropriate to occupational therapy, it has to be based on the assumptions of the profession. While occupational therapists will have to initially put time and energy into understanding a particular model, once they are familiar with it the structure of the model can usually be used to guide practice. That is, the assumptions underpinning the model become internalized and the person using it does not need to constantly refer to its assumptions each time they use it. Therefore models of practice essentially provide a "shortcut" for guiding professional reasoning. By using the model properly, professionals can have confidence they are faithful to the assumptions of the profession.

Second, models of practice help define the scope of practice. They have embedded within them assumptions about the domain of concern of occupational therapy. They shape the way professionals "see" their practice, and they provide guidance about what falls within the scope of practice and what does not. They provide a focus for the occupational therapist and define the parameters of factors and information that should be included in the planning of assessment and intervention. Some models provide specific guidance through the development of assessments that deal specifically with the model's concepts. Occupational therapists are guided to pay particular attention to those issues that are within the scope of their practice and to know when other professionals or services might best deal with other matters.

Third, models of practice can enhance professionalism and accountability. Three criteria form the basis for claims of professional status: (1) an independent body of knowledge and expertise, with a university degree as a minimum standard of education; (2) recognition of professional status at a state (government) level; and (3) self-regulation (autonomy) through ethical decision-making guided by a code of ethics (Williams and Lawlis 2019). In making explicit the theoretical assumptions of the profession upon which they are based, models of practice contribute to this demonstration of an independent body of knowledge.

Professions need to be accountable and critically review their professional knowledge base and make it publicly available. Models of practice are a way that the profession makes its knowledge base explicit and can contribute to the critical review of that knowledge base. The historical approach we take in this book emphasizes this function of models by discussing the reasons for their development and any perceived gap in the profession's discourse that the model aimed to fill.

Fourth, models of practice assist occupational therapists to be systematic and comprehensive in their collection of information. Occupational therapy models aim to guide occupational therapists to develop a holistic understanding of their clients. Each aims to set out a holistic theoretical framework (as the authors see it at the time of the model's development or revision), which can be used to assist occupational therapists to avoid some of the problems inherent in human reasoning. For example, it is acknowledged that clinical/professional reasoning is affected by a number of factors, including the order in which information is obtained. Humans tend to favor the hypotheses they have developed and can tend to overemphasize information that supports a favored hypothesis and disregard information that does not support or refutes it. By using a model of practice, therapists can be guided to overcome a tendency to collect information according to routines and habits that are not comprehensive (or have "blind spots") and to be more systematic in the sources and type of information they collect. Models of practice can also help them identify gaps in their knowledge and actively seek out information they might not have, rather than being overly influenced by the information they have already acquired.

Finally, models of practice provide guidance about what could *ideally* be done. As stated, they are comprehensive and holistic. However, they also aim to guide practice beyond one particular practice or organizational setting. Because it is not possible for models to be context specific, they can be very useful in guiding occupational therapists to work out more "ideal" solutions. However, they cannot possibly account for the specific contexts in which individual therapists find themselves. Therefore it requires professional reasoning by occupational therapists to determine what can be done in that particular practice setting, given the constraints of factors such as time, resources, role expectations, and the skills of the therapist. Models can provide the logic on which these decisions can be made.

Conclusion

Professionals draw upon complex and extensive knowledge bases for their practice. As professionals are expected to be able to think and act in practice, these knowledge bases cover different types of knowledge that support different aspects of professional practice. Two of these types of knowledge are theory (episteme) and practical knowledge (phronesis). Professionals also have to use knowledge of themselves and their own skills and abilities.

A range of different terminology has been used to categorize theory in occupational therapy. Use of terms depends on the way different levels of theory are categorized by the author. This chapter reviewed some ways that terminology has been used to refer to theory and its relationship to practice. In this book we focus on models of practice, the level of theory that aims to guide practice. Models of practice aim to guide occupational therapists to put into action the profession's unique understanding of occupation and its relationship to everyday life.

Being able to put occupational therapy into action requires not only knowledge of the profession's unique perspective, but also an understanding of the context within which that action must take place and the ability to identify and choose from a range of potential actions. In this chapter we highlighted that occupational therapists work with particular people in specific contexts.

We also emphasized that, while models of practice aim to guide practice, occupational therapists are required to use their professional reasoning skills to make decisions in practice. As Kielhofner (1995) stated, "Theory can never tell therapists, in advance, exactly what should be done in the context of therapy" (p. 1). Models of practice provide a framework within which to reason, but occupational therapists also require the ability to reason and make decisions about action.

In Chapter 2 we explore professional reasoning in context and present the Model of Context-specific Professional Reasoning (or MCPR). This model provides a framework for exploring the contexts that shape the encounters between occupational therapists and their clients. The contexts of occupational therapists shape their roles and purposes and include the social, political, and organizational contexts in which they work. They also exist as members of their professional communities of practice. Models of practice are artifacts of this community and help occupational therapists determine their role within a particular organization and with particular clients. Because they are based in the philosophical perspectives of the profession, models of practice combine with professional reasoning to guide practitioners in determining how to be an occupational therapist in a particular context with particular clients and in combining thinking and action.

References

Aristotle. *The Nicomachean Ethics*, Books I–X. Ross D, trans. Oxford University Press: 1975.

Chaparro C, Ranka J. Clinical reasoning in occupational therapy. In: Higgs J, Jenson GM, Loftus S, Christensen N, eds. *Clinical Reasoning in the Health Professions*. 4th ed. Elsevier; 2019:271–283.

Cohn ES, Coster WJ. Examining how theory guides practice: theory and practice in occupational therapy. In: Crepeau EB, Cohn ES, Boyt Schell BA, eds. *Willard & Spackman's Occupational Therapy*. 11th ed. Lippincott Williams & Wilkins; 2019:584–600.

Cole MB, Tufano R. *Applied Theories in Occupational Therapy: A Practical Approach*. Slack; 2008.

Crepeau EB, Boyt Schell BA, Cohn E. Theory and practice in occupational therapy. In: Crepeau EB, Cohn ES, Boyt Schell BA, eds. *Willard & Spackman's Occupational Therapy*. 11th ed. Lippincott Williams & Wilkins; 2009:428–434.

Duncan EAS. An introduction to conceptual models of practice and frames of reference. In: Duncan EAS, ed. *Foundations for Practice in Occupational Therapy*. 6th ed. Elsevier; 2020:38–43.

Kessels JPAM, Korthagen FAJ. The relationship between theory and practice: back to the classics. *Educ Researcher*. 1996 Apr;25(3):17–22.

Kielhofner G. *A Model of Human Occupation: Theory and Application*. 2nd ed. Lippincott Williams & Wilkins; 1995.

Kielhofner G. *Conceptual Foundations of Occupational Therapy*. 4th ed. F.A. Davis; 2009.

Madsen J, Josephsson S. Engagement in occupation as an inquiring process: exploring the situatedness of occupation. *J Occup* Sci. 2017;24(4):412–424. doi:10.1080/14427591.2017.1308266

Mattingly C, Fleming MH. *Clinical Reasoning: Forms of Inquiry in a Therapeutic Practice*. F.A. Davis; 1994.

Mattingly C, Fleming MH. Action and narrative: two dynamics of clinical reasoning. In: Higgs J, Jenson GM, Loftus S, Christensen N, eds. *Clinical Reasoning in the Health Professions*. 4th ed. Elsevier; 2019:119–127.

Mosey AC. *Applied Scientific Inquiry in the Health Professions: An Epistemological Orientation*. American Occupational Therapy Association; 1992.

Reel K, Feaver S. Models – terminology and usefulness. In: Davis S, ed. *Rehabilitation: The Use of Theories and Models in Practice*. Churchill Livingstone; 2006:49–62.

Ryle G. *The Concept of Mind*. Penguin Books; 1949.

Sackett DL. *Evidence Based Medicine: How to Practice and Teach EBM*. Churchill Livingstone; 2000.

Turpin M, Hanson D. Learning professional reasoning in practice through fieldwork. In: Boyt Schell BA, Schell J, eds. *Clinical and Professional Reasoning in Occupational Therapy*. 3rd ed. Wolters Kluwer; 2023.

Turpin M, Higgs J. Clinical reasoning and EBP. In: Hoffman T, Bennett S, Bennett J, Del Mar C, eds. *Evidence-Based Practice Across the Health Professions*. Churchill Livingstone; 2010:300–317.

Williams L, Lawlis T. The sociology of allied health. In: Germov J, ed. *Second Opinion: An Introduction to Health Sociology*. 6th ed. Oxford University Press; 2019.

CHAPTER 2

Professional Reasoning in Context

CHAPTER CONTENTS

The Context of Professional Practice   23

Communities of Practice   25

Occupational Therapy Professional
Reasoning   26

Historical View of Professional Reasoning in
Occupational Therapy   26

Art, Science, and Action   28

A Model for Professional Reasoning in
Context   29

Foreground Features   31

Background Features   32

Occupational Therapy Reasoning in
Action   34

Occupational Therapy Professional
Reasoning and Models of Practice   34

Conclusion   36

References   37

Chapter 1 explored different types of knowledge associated with theory and practice that professionals need to combine to take reasoned action. The first type of knowledge, which is associated with theory, is generalized propositional knowledge. Also known as *declarative knowledge* or *episteme* and consistent with Ryle's (1949) concept of knowing *that*, it is the type of knowledge that can be transmitted in words and therefore is open to public scrutiny. The second type of knowledge, which aligns with practice, is nonpropositional knowledge. It involves practical wisdom or professional practice knowledge and is also referred to as *procedural knowledge, phronesis,* and knowing *how*. It is context-specific knowledge that relates to specific people and places. As practitioners gain experience, their practice knowledge becomes embodied and is often difficult to put into words. This type of knowledge also includes practitioners' personal knowledge; that is, their knowledge of themselves as people: their personality, values and beliefs, preferences, and skills and challenges. Both types of knowledge are used in occupational therapy practice.

In this chapter we further explore the process of taking reasoned action. A process of reasoning is required to make decisions about action. The process of making professional decisions occurs within specific contexts, and the information occupational therapists seek as a basis for their professional decision-making is shaped by both the profession's domain of concern and the organizational, sociopolitical, and cultural contexts within which they work. To better understand how occupational therapists navigate the process of making professional decisions in context, we refer to the literature on clinical and professional reasoning. We present professional practice as a complex endeavor that requires judgment and critical reasoning, has ethical and practical dimensions, requires the logical use of "facts" and generalized theoretical principles as well as compassion and self-knowledge, and occurs within the context of various communities of professional and organizational practice. Regarding terminology, throughout this chapter we use the terms *clinical and professional reasoning* and *professional reasoning* to denote the reasoning that occupational therapists use in their professional role. We have chosen not to use the term *clinical reasoning*, in acknowledgment that occupational therapy practice is broader than simply a clinical venture (except when we present the historical literature on clinical reasoning, for which this term is accurate).

This chapter is organized according to the argument that the context of professional practice requires use of a professional knowledge base when engaged in professional reasoning and making decisions in practice, and that frameworks can be used to guide this professional reasoning in practice. First we explore the context of professional practice in terms of both the trait approach to professions and the communities of practice in which occupational therapists learn, work, and develop expertise. Then we look at occupational therapy practice in terms of professional reasoning. We present a historical account outlining how the clinical and professional reasoning of occupational therapists has been investigated, and we explore occupational therapy's unique practice in terms of art, science, and action. Next, we propose the Model of Context-specific Professional Reasoning (MCPR) as a framework for conceptualizing occupational therapy practice. We round out the chapter with a discussion of the role of occupational therapy practice models in supporting clinical and professional reasoning.

The Context of Professional Practice

Occupational therapy is an important profession in society. Therefore we commence our investigation of occupational therapy practice by considering the nature of professional practice more generally, beginning with the question: what does it mean to be a professional? According to the trait approach, which uses a structural functionalist perspective, professions need to meet four criteria for professional status (Williams and Lawlis 2019): (1) an independent body of knowledge and expertise, (2) a university degree as a minimum requirement, (3) state recognition of professional status, and (4) self-regulation through a code for ethical decision-making.

With professional status come certain rights and obligations. These rights include higher levels of financial remuneration and greater autonomy, for which society expects a higher level of expertise. This obligation for expertise relates to both skills and knowledge, in that professions often claim certain skills as exclusive to that profession and each profession must demonstrate a particular and extensive knowledge base that others in society would not normally be expected to possess.

Professionals practicing within a profession are afforded a level of autonomy, in that they are expected to fulfill their societal functions without having to detail everything they do and think. Because their reasoning is expected to be based on their extensive and unique knowledge base, it follows that only others who share that same knowledge base can fully understand what is required of and appropriate to that profession. Therefore professions are expected to engage in self-regulation.

Professions demonstrate their trustworthiness to undertake their roles in society through the development of codes of ethics. These are statements of the types of behaviors that can be expected of members of that profession. Often, professionals have access to privileged and sensitive information and they need to be able to assure society that they will deal with this information properly. For example, in the context of the helping professions, clients often disclose very personal information about themselves to professionals and might need to participate in activities that require closer contact than they would ordinarily have with people (such as having a person they don't know very well toilet or shower them). Therefore the codes of ethics of the helping professions detail the nature of the relationships in which professionals will and will not engage, how the rights of people receiving services will be upheld and protected, and how people's information will be handled. Consequently, codes of ethics usually contain statements about respecting clients and their privacy, maintaining relationships that have appropriate boundaries and that acknowledge the power imbalance inherent in professional relationships, and providing competent and effective services.

The purpose of codes of ethics is associated with the autonomy afforded to and self-regulation expected of professions. While codes of ethics are necessary for outlining the behaviors that society should be able to expect from professionals, they also provide the foundation for self-regulation. The reputation of a profession is dependent on the degree to which the behaviors outlined in these codes are adhered to by individual professionals and the support for professional standards that is provided by regulatory bodies.

Another distinguishing feature of professional practice is the expectation that professionals can use judgment to determine the best course of action in any given situation. As professionals are asked to deal with complex situations and problems, they are expected to use their judgment to discern *when* to apply *which* procedures (and when to refrain from applying them). Often, the ability to use a high level of judgment is the criterion that distinguishes professionals from technicians, in that technicians might have a high level of technical expertise but not the knowledge base required to make complex judgments. For professional practice, it is necessary but not sufficient to have only the technical skills required to carry out a range of procedures. Professionals are expected to use their extensive knowledge to respond to a variety of problems that present in different situations.

The primary purpose of this expert judgment is to make decisions about a course of action. Carr (1995) emphasized that professional action is not "right" in an absolute sense (of there being a right thing to do) but that it is right when it is "*reasoned* action that can be defended discursively in argument and justified as morally appropriate to the particular circumstances in which it was taken" (p. 71, italics in original). More recently, Higgs and Jensen (2019) explained that clinical reasoning (or professional judgment) involves the following three types of action: "*wise action*, meaning taking the best judged action in a specific context...; *professional action* encompassing ethical, accountable and self-regulatory decisions and conduct; and *person-centred action* that demonstrates respect for and collaboration with clients, caregivers and colleagues" (p. 3). Thus the purpose of using professional judgment is to determine action that is reasoned, wise, professional, and client centered.

Given that professionals are expected to possess extensive theoretical knowledge, making professional judgments in practice about appropriate action has traditionally been conceptualized as a process of *applying* theory. However, this assumption has been questioned. Many years ago, Mattingly and Fleming (1994) stated of occupational therapists:

> *While [they] sometimes speak of clinical reasoning as the application of theory to practice, this is a deceptive statement. A grounding in theory is essential for expert practice but does not guarantee such practice. One cannot do without such grounding, but it, alone, will not yield good clinical interventions, because theoretical reasoning differs from practical reasoning. (p. 9.)*

If, as Mattingly and Fleming (1994) argued, theory is essential for professional practice but insufficient to guarantee expert practice, professionals might need a range of different types of knowledge and skills to support their practice. As professionals need to both make judgments about and engage in reasoned action, they need information that supports them to gain an expert understanding of the overall situation as well as information that provides the basis for judgments about action.

The different types of knowledge that we discussed in Chapter 1 are necessary for expert and well-reasoned professional practice. By understanding the general principles conveyed through propositional knowledge, professionals can generate an understanding of specific situations from a broader perspective (e.g., using knowledge bases such as anatomy, physiology, psychology, and sociology). They have knowledge of the general effectiveness of certain interventions, using "evidence" generated from systematic research such as randomized controlled trials, and the perspective generated by their specific profession's theories. However they also need nonpropositional knowledge (professional practice knowledge and personal knowledge). Context-specific professional practice knowledge underpins their ability to judge what action is required in that specific situation and to know how to carry out that action. Personal knowledge is used for the interpersonal aspects of professional action because the ability to listen to, communicate with, and develop a professional relationship with clients and to regulate one's own behavior is well recognized as an essential component of professional practice (Taylor 2019; Turpin and Copley 2023).

In summary, to be a professional means to fulfill a social role. This comes with social expectations as well as social privileges. The expectations include ethically sound behavior and the ability to make well-reasoned and thoughtful judgments about action. These expert judgments are expected to be based on a unique and extensive foundation of propositional knowledge. It is increasingly recognized that well-reasoned judgments also rely on nonpropositional knowledge such as professional practice knowledge and personal knowledge.

Communities of Practice

While professional practice is situated within a society that expects its professionals to be able to provide unique services, it also exists within the historical and social contexts of a particular profession. Many years ago, Carr (1995) explained that to practice as a professional "is always to act within a tradition, and it is only by submitting to its authority that practitioners can begin to acquire the practical knowledge and standards of excellence by means of which their own practical competence can be judged" (pp. 68–69).

Professionals are expected to develop expertise or practical wisdom in a specific type of practice, but how does this occur? A traditional approach to this question is to focus on the knowledge and skills that characterize the practice of the profession. From this perspective, teaching students and novice professionals the knowledge and skills of the profession is the logical approach to the development of expertise. The structure of many professional courses requires students to demonstrate their acquisition of the knowledge base that underpins practice as well as those skills deemed necessary for that kind of practice. In addition, practice educators recognize the importance of practical experience in developing expertise (Evenson and Hanson 2019). Consequently, bodies such as the World Federation of Occupational Therapists outline what they conceive as minimum standards for professional education that include a minimum number of hours of practice-based learning (World Federation of Occupational Therapists 2016). Professional expertise is based on practical experience as well as the acquisition of knowledge and skills.

Sociocultural approaches to learning provide a useful way of explaining the development of professional expertise. These approaches emphasize that learning is situated within particular social contexts and cultures. In their seminal work, Lave and Wenger (1991) used the term *communities of practice* (p. 29) to refer to the communities to which individuals belong and within which they engage in situated or context-specific learning. Individual professionals develop expertise by participating in the cultural practices of the community of practice (this could refer to the profession of occupational therapy and the multidisciplinary teams in which occupational therapists work). Cultural practices include actions that are accepted as routine within a particular group. Often, such practices are so accepted and routine that they are no longer noticed by the group. They are often described as tacit or embedded in practice because they are not generally put into words or commented on.

From this perspective, professional learning is not simply the acquisition of skills and knowledge but involves a transformation in the way individuals participate in their communities of practice. This process of transformation is a mutual one; as people participate in their community of practice, they become enculturated within it, and their participation also changes the community's practices.

Participation in cultural practices contributes to a transformation in the identity and action of the professional. Similarly, such participation results in a transformation in practices, which contributes to the growth and development of the profession. The historical approach taken in this book demonstrates how occupational therapy models have changed over time and reveals something of the transformation that has occurred in the profession of occupational therapy through various authors' participation in the scholarly community of practice.

Professional relationships are important for learning cultural practices. As Kauffman (2019) stated, "A central tenet of situated learning is that learning occurs through social interaction. It emphasises-that learning is a co-construction through the interaction with and bonds between members of the community." (p. 51.) Through participation and engagement in the activity and discourse of the community, people learn about its values and shared knowledge and practices, what is expected, and how things are done. Learners engage with a range of different members of the community of practice, including supervisors, mentors, experts, and peers. Learning can be scaffolded, with the higher levels of support provided to novice learners being gradually reduced as they demonstrate their ability to contribute to the community of practice. In occupational therapy, Turpin et al. (2020) described how one occupational therapy department provided a community of practice for newly graduated occupational therapists. Experienced occupational therapists used a process of guided questioning to support the new graduates to develop their clinical and professional reasoning skills. Over a few months, as the new graduates became more proficient in using this questioning process themselves, they did not require this higher level of support for their clinical and professional reasoning, and it was reduced. As professionals, they needed to be able to independently use their clinical and professional reasoning skills to guide their assessment and intervention and make decisions in practice.

Occupational Therapy Professional Reasoning

Now we turn to an exploration of clinical and professional reasoning in occupational therapy. Occupational therapy professional reasoning is central to decisions about action. As professionals, occupational therapists need to be able to make well-reasoned decisions about their professional action under conditions of uncertainty (Turpin and Higgs 2017). It is through a process of professional reasoning that occupational therapists make decisions about the information to gather to understand their clients' situations, histories, and life goals and dreams. It is through professional reasoning that they make decisions about interventions to achieve outcomes that are meaningful for their clients. In this section we discuss developments in occupational therapy professional reasoning from a historical perspective; explore the nature of occupational therapy practice as requiring art, science, and action; and propose a model for conceptualizing context-specific reasoning in occupational therapy.

HISTORICAL VIEW OF PROFESSIONAL REASONING IN OCCUPATIONAL THERAPY

In occupational therapy, research into the process of thinking and making judgments in practice has generally adopted the term *clinical reasoning*. This term was used in medicine, and the early conceptualizations of occupational therapy reasoning were largely influenced by that research. The initial clinical reasoning research in occupational therapy was conducted in the early 1980s (Rogers 1983; Rogers and Masagatani 1982). At that time, clinical reasoning was generally understood from the perspective of artificial intelligence, with its focus on acquiring and managing information. Therefore clinical reasoning was described as a process involving the acquisition and interpretation of *cues* or information, and the generation and testing of *hypotheses* about what the cues might mean and their implications for professional action. This way of thinking was called *hypothetico-deductive reasoning* because the emphasis was on using hypotheses to guide a logical and systematic process of collecting and combining information and deductively interpreting it in the light of hypotheses about potential meaning.

Research funded by the American Occupational Therapy Association (AOTA) and conducted by Mattingly and Fleming in the late 1980s has dominated subsequent thinking about clinical reasoning in occupational therapy. Mattingly and Fleming (1994) observed clinical practice in a large rehabilitation facility in the United States. They argued that reasoning could be categorized into four different types: (1) procedural, (2) interactive, (3) conditional, and (4) narrative. This work was influential, not only through the results of their methodologically rigorous research, but also through the introduction of the idea that occupational therapists might use multiple ways of reasoning. Prior to their work, clinical reasoning in occupational therapy had been conceptualized only as a hypothetico-deductive process (i.e., in the same way as medicine). In contrast, Mattingly and Fleming stated that, in occupational therapy, "different modes of thinking are employed for different purposes and in response to particular features of the clinical problem complex" (p. 17).

Using the term *three-track mind*, Mattingly and Fleming (1994; also see Fleming 1991) observed that occupational therapists switched among three modes of reasoning so rapidly that they appeared to be using them simultaneously. First they used procedural reasoning, which relates to situations in which therapists' reasoning centered on defining problems and considering intervention possibilities. They thought about the *procedures* they might use to remediate the problems a person was having with functional performance. Second, an interactive mode of reasoning was used when the therapist wanted to "interact with and better understand the person" (p. 17). This understanding appeared to be particularly important when the therapist wanted to tailor their intervention for a specific client. The third mode of reasoning that formed part of the three-track mind was conditional reasoning. This is "a complex form of social reasoning, [which] is used to help the patient in the difficult process of reconstructing a life that is now permanently changed by injury or disease" (p. 17). In their discussion of this mode of reasoning, Mattingly and Fleming associated it with experienced occupational therapists and alluded to the problems of putting language to an aspect of practice that is largely unspoken. They wrote, "The concept of conditional reasoning is perhaps the most elusive notion in our proposed theory of multiple modes of thinking. Yet we are firmly, if intuitively, convinced that there is a third form of reasoning that many experienced therapists used. This reasoning style moves beyond specific concerns about the person and the physical problems and places them in broader social and temporal contexts." (p. 18.) In addition to the three modes of reasoning that contributed to the three-track mind, the final form of reasoning these authors proposed was a narrative mode of reasoning, in which occupational therapists swapped stories and engaged others in discussing puzzling situations. They suggested that this storytelling also served to enlarge participants' "fund of practical knowledge" vicariously (p. 18).

In 1993, Schell and Cervero published an "integrative review" of the clinical reasoning literature at the time. A range of terms had been used to discuss a hypothetico-deductive approach to clinical reasoning, such as *diagnostic reasoning* (Rogers 1983) and *procedural reasoning* (Mattingly 1991; Mattingly and Fleming 1994), and Schell and Cervero grouped these together and labeled the category *scientific reasoning*. This term was adopted by other authors and was used frequently in subsequent publications relating to clinical reasoning in occupational therapy. Possibly taking Mattingly and Fleming's lead of proposing that occupational therapists use multiple modes of reasoning, Schell and Cervero proposed an additional category of reasoning, which they called *pragmatic reasoning*. Pragmatic reasoning referred to those times when occupational therapists thought about what *could* be done, given the practice resources available in the situation, the broader organizational and political context, and the wishes of the client. They also referred to *ethical reasoning*, where occupational therapists attended to what *should* be done (Rogers 1983).

These earlier studies were followed by a continued interest in clinical reasoning over the following years, with several journals publishing special editions on clinical reasoning in the mid-1990s. Subsequently, Unsworth (2005) undertook research to test the presence of the various types of reasoning that had been described. She concluded that occupational therapists do appear to use procedural, interactive, conditional, and pragmatic reasoning (proposing that pragmatic reasoning was more related to the influence of the practice environment than to the therapist's personal philosophy) and that occupational therapists also seemed to use a process of linking the current situation to broader principles. She called this process *generalization reasoning* and presented it as a subcategory of each of the other types of reasoning. Examples of generalization reasoning included generalizing about people with a particular medical diagnosis and general principles relating to the provision of services (both in that organization or service context and relating more specifically to occupational therapy interventions). She likened this process of generalizing from the client and then focusing back on them to using a zoom lens on a camera. The process occurred very rapidly.

This historical journey through clinical reasoning literature and research in occupational therapy demonstrates that the concept was initially framed and approached as it had been in medicine. The subsequent work of Mattingly and Fleming provided a pivotal point for a new understanding of clinical reasoning in occupational therapy. This work prompted the occupational therapy profession to see itself with fresh eyes. The following section explores occupational therapy's unique perspective toward the notions of art and science and presents action as a primary feature of occupational therapy clinical reasoning.

Art, Science, and Action

When discussing the complexity of practice, Mattingly and Fleming (1994) observed that occupational therapy was a profession between two cultures: the culture of biomedicine and its own professional culture. As they stated, "one of the most interesting features of occupational therapy practice is that it tends to deal with functional problems that fall nicely within biomedicine (treating physical injuries with specific treatment techniques), as well as problems going far beyond the physical body, encompassing social, cultural, and psychological issues that concern the meaning of illness or injury to a person's life" (p. 37). In labeling this observation, they referred to occupational therapy as a "two-body practice" (p. 37), whereby occupational therapists attend to both physical and phenomenological bodies.

While different professions attend to each perspective to various degrees (e.g., medicine and physiotherapy predominantly focus on the body, and social work generally attends to clients' experiences and the social structures that shape them), Mattingly and Fleming (1994) presented occupational therapists as seemingly unique among the health professions by attending to both features equally. In 2005 Blair and Robertson claimed that occupational therapy lies on "what might be considered to be a 'professional fault line' between health and social care" (p. 272), whereby they seemed to be equating healthcare with a scientific, biomedical approach and social care with a perspective more concerned with people's social and personal welfare. This dual orientation strongly contributes to the complexity of reasoning required in occupational therapy.

The process required for such dual attention has long been referred to in occupational therapy using the concepts of art and science. A familiar definition of occupational therapy refers to the "art and science of man's [sic] participation..." (AOTA 1972, p. 204). The equal importance of both perspectives was emphasized by Turpin (2007), who stated, "When occupational therapists refer to the paired concepts of art and science, they express their moral dissatisfaction with being constrained by either. In isolation, art somehow seems too soft and unquantifiable and science too hard and unyielding. The pairing of art and science expresses the complexity of occupational therapy; we are not one thing, but many" (p. 482). Occupational therapists need to be able to manage and balance these two perspectives in a way that enables them to act with both competence and care.

The importance of art and science to occupational therapy can be seen in its valuing of different types of evidence to support practice. For example, both quantitative and qualitative research is used to build occupational therapy's knowledge base. Quantitative research is often used to evaluate the effectiveness of interventions and formal evaluation tools. Quantitative research is often used to explore people's experiences and the phenomenological aspects of life.

Also contributing to an understanding of occupational therapy's complexity is the observation that action, observation, and interpretation are integral to occupational therapy reasoning. Mattingly and Fleming (1994) observed that occupational therapists don't just reason and then act, but reason *through* action and observation. For example, to collect or interpret information, they ask their clients to do certain things while observing them and engage in action themselves. The information they collect helps them understand how people are performing their everyday occupations. This understanding then informs further action to collect more specific information or to test their judgments about interventions or their understanding of the situation.

Reasoning in action is not simply a process of trial and error, but a specific and targeted process. Mattingly and Fleming (1994) concluded that occupational therapists compare their observations with their preexisting "stock of basic knowledge" (p. 322) when making interpretations and inferences. As they stated, "observations become information only if they can be used against a backdrop of prior knowledge" (p. 322). It may be that the process Unsworth (2005) called "generalization reasoning" is the same as the linking of observations made in specific situations to a stock of prior knowledge. Both types of knowledge discussed in Chapter 1, propositional and nonpropositional knowledge, can contribute to this stock of prior knowledge. As occupational therapists gain experience, learning from these experiences is added to this stock of knowledge. This explains why expert occupational therapists form their judgments based on "smaller bits of information" (Mattingly and Fleming 1994, p. 323) and less but more targeted action than novice occupational therapists. They have a more extensive (and probably more organized) stock of knowledge from which to draw when planning action. Thus the process of reasoning in action becomes more refined as occupational therapists' stocks of knowledge expand through increased experience and knowledge (through, for example, continuing professional development activities and reading professional journals) and they can compare their action with increasingly relevant knowledge.

A Model for Professional Reasoning in Context

Occupational therapists reason and make decisions in specific contexts. As we have discussed, professional reasoning is needed to determine what to do with a specific client, and occupational therapists use a process of reasoning in action to collect and interpret information and make practice decisions. The Model of Context-specific Professional Reasoning (MCPR) provides a framework for conceptualizing how occupational therapists reason in practice and the contextual features that shape their reasoning. The MCPR conceptualizes professional reasoning as highly contextualized. It highlights that encounters between clients (whether individuals or collectives) and therapists occur within broader organizational, legislative, policy, and cultural contexts and are shaped by the perspectives each person brings to the encounter and the relationship that is developed between them.

Fig. 2.1 is a diagrammatic representation of the MCPR. The model centers on the encounter between occupational therapists and specific people against a background of context. This emphasizes that professional reasoning is ultimately context and person specific. The diagram also includes the reasoning-in-action process.

The choice of the word *person(s)* might appear to invite criticism that the model only applies to work with individual clients, but this is not the case. The term *person* was purposely selected

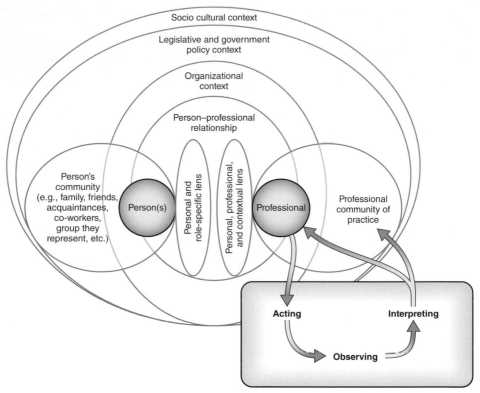

Fig. 2.1   Model of Context-specific Professional Reasoning.

over *client* because the model distinguished between the *focus* of the work (which often relates to clients) and the *interaction* with specific people. Regarding the focus of the work, clients can include large and small groups or collectives of individuals as well as individuals and formal entities. For example, occupational therapists might work with individual clients and their families, groups of individuals, or entities such as organizations (e.g., government and nongovernment agencies) and companies (e.g., those seeking to increase the safety of their employees). In some cases, the groups at which occupational therapists target their work are whole populations or subpopulations (in such cases, these collectives are not generally referred to as *clients*). For example, an occupational therapist might be advocating for or engaged in developing policy that will provide needed resources to facilitate the participation of individuals with a disability (where they are working with images of the types of people who would have access to resources and would benefit from policy changes).

Regardless of where the work is focused, it requires the professional to *interact* with certain people. These people might be the clients themselves, people who have concerns for or connections with individual clients, or people who represent or are responsible for others in formal organizations such as an agency or corporation. The ultimate purpose of this interaction is for the professional to engage in action directly or to facilitate the action of others.

Regardless of whether occupational therapists are working directly with individuals, with groups of individuals, or through larger entities and collectives, they aim to make a positive impact upon the health, well-being, and participation of specific people—whether those people can be identified individually or are just seen as part of a larger group, entity, or population. For example, an occupational therapist might be working with Mary Smith to improve their desired or needed participation in life roles by reducing impairments or finding new ways to conduct occupations or adapting aspects of their environment. Alternatively, the occupational therapist might be working on a population-based health promotion campaign with the aim of improving the lives of people *like* Mary Smith (i.e., the occupational therapist can't identify which specific persons will benefit from the project). With these examples in mind, we conceptualize professional reasoning as aiming to impact specific people. Therefore we have used the term *person* in the model to denote this.

Embedded within the model is the assumption that individuals exist within the context of relationships with others (both formal and informal). In that respect, the MCPR can be seen as influenced by a sociocultural approach. People live within broader social and cultural contexts. They are influenced by the people with whom they have direct relationships, larger communities of people and the ideas that are debated or taken for granted by those communities (often referred to as *culture* in its broader sense), and various ways the society in which they live is structured and organized. Generally, these sociocultural perspectives are internalized by people, who are often unaware of their influence.

The diagram of the model presents some of the contexts that surround the professional and the person(s) with whom they are interacting when developing or providing a service. To simplify discussion of this complex situation, the diagram is divided into a *foreground* and a *background*. In the foreground of the diagram are the professionals and persons who bring their own specific perspectives to the encounter. Borrowing from Schell (2009), these are represented in the diagram as "lenses." Surrounding each person engaged in the encounter is a particular community that also influences their perspectives. For both the person and the occupational therapist, these include the other people in their communities that influence their lives and perspectives. In addition, professionals are part of professional "communities of practice" (Lave and Wenger 1991).

In the background are various layers of social context that influence the encounter. In the diagram these are represented as (1) the person–professional relationship, which denotes the concept that relationships among people are more than the sum of the interactions by which they are constituted; (2) the organizational context, which aims to denote the particular practice environments in which the encounter occurs; (3) the context of legislation and policy that surrounds the encounter and within which all the key characters in the encounter live; and (4) the broader sociocultural context of the society.

Fig. 2.1 also includes a blue box with arrows, which makes explicit the reasoning-in-action process that occupational therapists have been observed to use. Each aspect of the diagram is discussed in more detail in the sections that follow.

FOREGROUND FEATURES

The foreground features of the MCPR relate to the professional encounter between an occupational therapist and a person. In most practice scenarios, occupational therapists and persons/clients engage in some sort of encounter organized around the provision of a specific service. These encounters can be with clients or with other people in relation to clients, such as relatives, organizational representatives, and other professionals working with the client. Both occupational therapists and the person(s) with whom they interact bring their own perspectives to the encounter. We describe these as lenses, with the lenses of both parties being influenced by their own personal perspectives, as well as the expectations derived from their various roles in the encounter. Therefore the MCPR conceptualizes the person with whom the professional interacts as seeing the encounter through their "personal and role-specific lens."

The personal lens refers to their own personal characteristics such as personality, beliefs and worldview, and biographical situation and history. The role-specific lens refers to the role(s) the person is playing in the encounter, such as client, carer, co-worker or organizational representative, or policy developer. For example, in occupational therapy scenarios, the people engaging in the encounter in the role of client will bring expectations related to that role. They might have certain expectations of the professional's level of expertise and the degree of collaboration that should occur. They will also have expectations about their own behavior as a client. These expectations of themselves and professionals will be informed by previous experiences, stories from others in their community, and sociocultural expectations.

The professionals' lenses are threefold, as follows: (1) their *personal lens* refers to their own personal characteristics such as personality, beliefs and worldview, and biographical situation and history, just as it does for the other person; (2) their *professional lens* refers to their identity and experience as a member of a particular profession (e.g., an occupational therapist) and the way they have internalized the values and beliefs of their professional community; and (3) their *contextual lens* refers to their understanding and experience of their particular role within a specific practice context and the culture of that practice context. Like the other people in the encounter, occupational therapists bring expectations about their own behavior and that of the people with whom they are interacting. In addition to their professional lens, which shapes their expectations of their own professional behavior and the unique occupational therapy perspective, the way they see the encounter will be shaped by their contextual lens, which is informed by expectations about what occupational therapists do in that organization.

Both the person and the professional are also influenced by their respective communities. In the case of people receiving services (clients), they will have a range of experiences and formal and informal relationships with the people connected to them. These will all influence the perspectives they bring to the encounter—both their personal perspective and their expectations relating to the role of client—and the degree to which they are likely to follow recommendations the professional might make. These relationships will also influence the personal and material resources available to clients and will impact what *can* be done (pragmatic reasoning regarding intervention/service delivery options). For example, the number of people a family's financial resources must support will impact whether services that carry a financial cost can be offered and how often the relevant family members can afford to attend the service (i.e., cost of service, transport, time off from work, etc.). An intervention for a disabled person living in a group home might need commitment from support workers to carry out or supervise what has been recommended. Any recommendations for changes to workplaces will need to be appropriate to the culture of the workplace (of management and workers) and the processes required to undertake their core business.

As with their clients, professionals are also surrounded by their own communities, which will influence their personal perspectives. In addition to this, they are part of communities of practice, such as the local, national, and international communities of occupational therapists, which influence their professional perspective. As a profession, occupational therapy has its own unique knowledge base, values, and perspectives that influence the perspectives each practitioner will bring to an encounter with clients. They influence what kinds of information they seek and how they collect it, how they interpret information, and what kinds of interventions and services they feel they can offer.

BACKGROUND FEATURES

The background features of the MCPR are the broader, multilayered context within which professional encounters occur. The model identifies four major layers of context that surround any encounter between professionals and the people with whom they work: (1) the person–professional relationship, (2) the organizational context, (3) the legislative and government policy context, and (4) the sociocultural context. These layers are nested in such a way as to denote their proximity to the encounter. The innermost, more proximal layers are more likely to be brought to conscious awareness by the people involved in the encounter. The outer layers will influence the encounter in ways that might not be noticed and are the source of assumptions that are often taken for granted by the parties to the encounter.

The first layer is the *person–professional relationship*, which is the relationship created among the people involved in the encounter. While each person will bring their own lens to the encounter, the relationships that develop among the people involved will also influence the process and outcome of the encounter. Relationship is specified as a particular background feature because the relationships that people develop can influence the decisions that can be made. For example, an occupational therapist working with a particular organizational client might have built a facilitatory relationship with a particular manager and have a high level of confidence that their recommendations will be implemented. However, if a new person steps into that organizational position, the recommendations the occupational therapist makes might differ because their confidence in the implementation of their recommendations might be different. Similarly, a client and an occupational therapist might have a difficult relationship, and a referral to another occupational therapist might result in a better outcome for the client.

The importance of relationships between professionals and clients is well recognized as affecting the outcome of their encounters (Taylor 2019). Examples of these person–professional relationships include relationships with individual clients and their significant others, with groups of clients, with people in management or supervisory positions who are responsible for a group of workers or the management practices of a company, and with elders or leaders of community groups. These relationships are central to occupational therapy philosophy, as occupational therapists aim to work *with* people rather than doing things *to* them. It is through these different types of relationships that they aim to influence the health and well-being of individuals, groups, and populations.

The next layer of context relates to the *organization* in which the person–professional interaction occurs. We have called it *organizational context* because most occupational therapy work is undertaken within a specific practice context. Whether the occupational therapist is being paid or doing the work in a voluntary capacity, they are usually either providing services directly through organizations or working with organizations to influence their provision of services and resources. We are using the term *organization* in a broad way to denote a range of different types of organizations, such as government and nongovernment agencies, corporations, service delivery organizations, and incorporated bodies.

Organizations are important to consider as a context in which the person–professional encounter occurs because they have a culture that influences *what* work is done and *how* it is done. This culture shapes occupational therapy practice at subconscious and conscious levels. That is, occupational therapists might develop routine ways of seeing and doing things in a specific context or they might be consciously aware of the constraints and demands that the practice environment places on their practice. Organizations are established for certain purposes, and it is expected that people working for or with them will be instrumental in fulfilling those purposes. Such expectations will help shape occupational therapists' contextual lenses. Similarly, clients and others will bring expectations about that organization regarding the type and quality of the services or assistance provided. These expectations form part of their role-specific lenses.

The next layer of context relates to the society in which the encounter takes place. Larger societies have formal *legislative and government processes* that determine the rules of that society. In parliamentary democracies, laws are made through acts of Parliament and enforced by legal processes (e.g., courts) and regulators, and by organizations such as police forces. Societies may also have subgroups, in which persons hold recognized positions and provide leadership and governance to the subgroup; an example is elders of an Indigenous group. Both professionals and the people they work with must abide by the laws of the society and will be influenced by the policies and subsequent services and practices developed and/or funded by the government.

The final layer, which influences all the layers within it, is the *culture* of the society. Cultural and subcultural beliefs and practices pervade the lives of people and influence their behavior. They also influence the expectations and social mores relating to relationships between professionals and clients, as well as the organizations that are developed and the laws and policies that are created. Cultural beliefs and practices are often held and enacted at a subconscious level, as people who have grown up in those cultural contexts will have internalized many values and beliefs. They become taken-for-granted assumptions. Often, people only become aware of those values and beliefs when they are confronted with situations that do not align with them. This might occur because of a particular event or circumstance, through moving from one culture to another, or when subcultural values do not align with those of the dominant culture or other subcultures.

Occupational Therapy Reasoning in Action

In addition to the multiple layers that surround person and professional, the MCPR includes a specific feature of occupational therapy reasoning: reasoning in action. This is presented in the box in the lower right of Fig. 2.1. This box is informed by Mattingly and Fleming's (1994) observations and interpretations of occupational therapy clinical reasoning. They emphasized that action is an integral part of occupational therapists' clinical reasoning and linked this to the profession's roots in the philosophical perspective of pragmatism (see the work of John Dewey, William James, and Charles Sanders-Pierce). Readers will note that reference to pragmatism is made in several models reviewed in this book.

Mattingly and Fleming (1994) noted that occupational therapists often reason through action—both their own and the action of others. The occupational therapists in their research asked their clients to do something so that they could observe, with precision, how the clients undertook the tasks. They also acted themselves, through assessment and intervention, and observed the outcomes and made judgments based on their interpretations of those observations. Mattingly and Fleming (1994) found that occupational therapists interpreted their observations by comparing them with their stock of theoretical and practice-based knowledge. This process of interpretation enabled them to make judgments about the clinical situation and to plan further action. The experience gained from these cycles of action, observation, and interpretation was added to the professional's stock of knowledge and became part of the information against which further cycles of action were interpreted.

In Fig. 2.1 the reasoning-in-action process of acting, observing, and interpreting is represented by the arrows in the lower right. The knowledge generated through this process can be used by the individual occupational therapist and shared with the professional community of practice. Individual occupational therapists use this information to either make decisions or plan further cycles of action, observation, and interpretation. Sharing with others in the profession frequently occurs through informal and formal conversations and presentations with colleagues. The information and learning can also be shared more broadly with the professional community of practice through forums, professional magazines, conferences, and when undertaken as a formal part of research, in professional journals.

Occupational Therapy Professional Reasoning and Models of Practice

The MCPR highlights the complexity of factors that influence professional reasoning. These factors can relate to the personal, role-specific, professional, and contextual lenses that people bring to a professional encounter. They are shaped by the person–professional relationships that are developed; organizational, legislative, and government policies; and sociocultural contexts in which person–professional encounters occur. All these factors interact to create a unique situation for every person–professional encounter. The MCPR provides occupational therapists with a framework for considering these complex and unique factors when reflecting on their professional reasoning. See Box 2.1 for an example of an occupational therapist using the MCPR to analyse their professional reasoning.

BOX 2.1 ■ Reflecting on Professional Reasoning Using the MCPR

Claire is an occupational therapist with 10 years professional experience working with children with burns. She has recently joined a group of colleagues who meet monthly to discuss cases. Claire joined the group to keep her professional skills and knowledge up to date and to learn from the experience of others, given that she works as a sole occupational therapist in her department and craves more occupational therapy support. She is preparing to present one of her cases at the next meeting. She is using the MCPR to analyse her own experience and make explicit the factors that have influenced her reasoning in practice.

Her client, Matthew, is a one-year-old boy who was referred to occupational therapy after suffering severe burns at home. Matthew´s family left their home country because it was unsafe for them to stay there. They had to leave everything and now they live in impoverished conditions in their new country. Matthew is the youngest of four siblings, all of whom are under 10 years of age, and his mother works as a casual cleaner. Recently, his mother was holding him while cooking over an open flame. She had been drinking, as she often did to cope with her difficult life. While she was cooking, Matthew slipped from her arms and fell into the flames, sustaining burns to his face, upper limbs and chest.

Claire used the MCPR to reflect on her experience with Matthew. She thought that his case would be particularly interesting to the group because her decisions regarding Matthew´s care differed in many respects from those she usually made for other clients. In terms of the foreground components of the model, Clair needed to consider the person/s she was interacting with – their perspectives and circumstances. She has been seeing Matthew since he was admitted to hospital and has developed a strong bond with him. In contrast, she finds it difficult to connect with his mother, who seems quite distant and does not appear to interact with Matthew very much either. Claire has decided to make splints to avoid contractures in Matthew´s elbows and to reduce scaring by prescribing compression garments for his face, chest and arms. However, she knows that Matthew's mother has no experience of the healthcare system in her new country and doesn't know what is expected in the client/family role. Therefore, Claire is worried that Matthew's mother might not wash the garments regularly enough or misplace them, so she has organised to provide extra garments. Claire also has made sure that she writes down the instructions for wearing the splints and compression garments, adding drawings to make them clearer for his mother. Once a week she continues to phone Matthew's mother to encourage her to follow his wearing regime.

The MCPR foreground also prompted her to reflect on her own perspectives and context. Claire identified that her reasoning has been shaped by her community of practice and her professional lens, as well as the expectations of her context. Reflecting on her community of practice, Claire knew that she had decided to make splints and provide pressure garments because these are accepted occupational therapy interventions in this area of practice. She also knows that, while she tries to stay up to date with the current evidence for interventions in burns, her time and access to databases is limited. As an occupational therapist, she knew to consider Matthew´s young age, his deprived socio-cultural background, and the extent of the injuries he had sustained. Claire also considered his mother's low educational level. These factors influenced her reasoning in terms of providing more garments and additional support. Claire also knew that her decisions were shaped by her personal lens. She felt strongly for babies with burn injuries, knowing that they would have to endure interventions for many years. She was particularly sensitive regarding neglected or mistreated children because, when she was a child, she was physically and psychologically abused and neglected by her own parents.

In terms of the MCPR background, Claire first considered her relationship with Matthew and his mother. While she had a close bond with Matthew, she found his mother very difficult to connect with. Consequently, she had worked hard to ensure that his mother was engaged with his care and had support in her difficult circumstances. Regarding the organisational context, the intervention strategies she chose were a standard part of care in her workplace and were covered by the national health insurance. However, to provide more than the standard number of garments, she knew she had to seek special permission. She also needed to be aware of the laws and obligations for reporting suspected child abuse and neglect and to be aware of the sociocultural barriers facing Matthew's mother. Claire was surprised by the many factors that the MCPR guided her to identify as shaping her reasoning in practice.

An important aspect of the MCPR is the professional community of practice, which can be discipline specific or can comprise multi/transdisciplinary teams. As discussed earlier in the chapter, professionals develop their understanding of their professional discipline through professional socialization into communities of practice and the acquisition of the specific knowledge base unique to each profession. Professionals maintain their professional identities through access to and identification with their community of practice. This may involve direct contact with other members of the community of practice formally through workshops and special interest groups and informally through contact with co-workers. Less formal activities include reading publications produced by members of the community of practice and identifying with that community by working with members of other professions and defining oneself as an occupational therapist.

As professionals become socialized into their communities of practice, the values and perspectives of their professional group become internalized. Trede and Higgs (2008) explained that, as professional beliefs and values become increasingly embodied, they often become taken for granted and awareness of them decreases because they "represent the unquestioned norm" (p. 32) of their professional group. They cautioned that, unless they can make these assumptions overt, these norms can be difficult to examine and critique. Without such examination, the value of such norms cannot be established, either positively or negatively.

Conceptual models of practice provide a way that a shared vision of the occupational therapy community of practice is available and therefore open to public scrutiny. Each model of practice discussed in this book presents a particular way of organizing and describing occupational therapy's theoretical assumptions and values (the shared vision) for the purpose of guiding practice. They all share the perspectives and values that characterize occupational therapy as a profession and distinguish it from other professions. Therefore the core of occupational therapy is encapsulated within the commonalities of the models. However, each model also emphasizes different aspects of the shared vision to different degrees. This variation probably relates to a combination of the different practice environments for which some of the models were originally developed, sociocultural differences relating to the country in which or for which they were developed, the time in occupational therapy's history in which they were developed or revised, and the philosophical perspectives the authors chose to present or emphasize.

The chapters that follow present 11 occupational therapy conceptual models of practice. They were all developed to guide practice by providing a systematic way to organize many of the core concepts of occupational therapy. The advantage of using conceptual models to guide practice is that they provide a systematic and comprehensive way to conceptualize practice. Often, they are used in conjunction with other frameworks, which mostly provide greater detail about interventions and techniques relevant to a particular practice area. As discussed in Chapter 1, these are often referred to as *frames of reference* and frequently contain information that is not specific to occupational therapy. Conceptual models of practice, however, are specific to occupational therapy and contain the profession's core concepts. For each model, we describe its core concepts and an overview of its history, and provide a memory aid to facilitate use of the model in practice. We also provide the major references for each model. Because this book aims to give an *overview* of occupational therapy conceptual models of practice, readers are encouraged to develop a more in-depth understanding of the models they feel are most relevant to their own practices by accessing the texts in which they are presented by the authors.

Conclusion

In this chapter we discussed the nature of professional practice. We explored occupational therapy as a profession that requires a unique knowledge base and code of ethics, and that must engage in self-regulation. Professionals are expected to fulfill roles in society. They generally work under conditions of uncertainty and are required to engage in professional reasoning to make judgments about what action(s) to take in a particular circumstance. In their practice, occupational therapists are surrounded by a community of practice that provides professional socialization into the culture of occupational therapy. This community supports occupational therapists to learn to use professional reasoning and make appropriate decisions about what to do in practice. The community also maintains the professional knowledge base.

We also discussed two unique aspects of occupational therapy. First, occupational therapists value both art and science in equal measure in their understanding of the needs of clients and their expectations about the interventions or services they can offer. They place equal value on both when making decisions about what to do in their professional role.

Second, action is central to occupational therapy practice and an integral part of occupational therapists' professional reasoning and decision-making. That is, they often think in and through action, using a process of reasoning in action. Reasoning and decisions about action always occur within specific contexts, which shape and are shaped by these decisions and actions. Thus occupational therapy reasoning and decision-making are always context based. We presented the MCPR as a model for understanding the context-specific nature of occupational therapy professional reasoning. The MCPR explores the varying perspectives that occupational therapists and the people with whom they work bring to their professional encounters. It considers four layers of context that impact occupational therapists' professional reasoning. It also makes explicit the reasoning-in-action process used by occupational therapists.

One of the ways the occupational therapy community of practice makes its perspectives and practices clear is through models of practice. These models are a level of theory that specifically aims to guide practice. In the chapters that follow we present 11 occupational therapy models of practice. For each we present the major concepts as outlined in their most recent form, a discussion of their historical development, a list of major publications (these are not meant to be exhaustive but to provide a starting point for readers who wish to investigate the model in more detail), and a memory aid and case illustration to assist occupational therapists when using the model in their practice.

References

AOTA. Occupational therapy: Its definition and function. *Am J Occup Ther*. 1972 26:204

Blair SEE, Robertson L. Hard complexities – soft complexities: an exploration of philosophical positions related to evidence in occupational therapy. *Br J Occup Ther*. 2005 Jun 1;68(6):269–276.

Carr W. *For Education: Towards Critical Educational Inquiry*. The Open University; 1995.

Evenson M, Hanson D. Fieldwork, practice education, and professional entry. In: Boyt Schell BA, Gillen G, eds. *Willard & Spackman's Occupational Therapy*. 13th ed. Wolters Kluwer; 2019:1078–1099.

Fleming MH. The therapist with the three-track mind. *Am J Occup Ther*. 1991 Nov;45(11):1007–1014. doi:10.5014/ajot.45.11.1007

Higgs J, Jensen GM. Clinical reasoning: challenges of interpretation and practice in the 21st century. In: Higgs J, Jenson GM, Loftus S, Christensen N, eds. *Clinical Reasoning in the Health Professions*. 4th ed. Elsevier; 2019:3–12.

Kauffman DM. Teaching and learning in medical education: how theory can inform practice. In: Swanwick T, Forrest K, O'Brien BC, ed. *Understanding Medical Education: Evidence, Theory and Practice*. 3rd ed. Wiley Blackwell; 2019:37–69.

Lave J, Wenger E. *Situated Learning: Legitimate Peripheral Participation*. Cambridge University Press; 1991.

Mattingly C. The narrative nature of clinical reasoning. *Am J Occup Ther*. 1991 Nov;45(11): 998–1005. doi:10.5014/ajot.45.11.998

Mattingly C, Fleming MH. *Clinical Reasoning: Forms of Inquiry in a Therapeutic Practice*. F.A. Davis; 1994.

Rogers JC. Clinical reasoning: the ethics, science, and art. *Am J Occup Ther*. 1983 Sep;37(9):601–616. doi:10.5014/ajot.37.9.601

Rogers JC, Masagatani G. Clinical reasoning of occupational therapists during the initial assessment of physically disabled patients. *Occup Ther J Res*. 1982;2:195–219. doi:10.1177/153944928200200401

Ryle G. *The Concept of Mind*. Penguin Books; 1949.

Schell B. Professional reasoning in practice. In: Crepeau EB, Cohn ES, Boyt Schell BA, eds. *Willard & Spackman's Occupational Therapy*. 11th ed. Lippincott Williams & Wilkins; 2009:314–327.

Schell B, Cervero R. Clinical reasoning in occupational therapy: an integrative review. *Am J Occup Ther*. 1993 Jul;47(7):605–610. doi:10.5014/ajot.47.7.605

Taylor RR. Therapeutic relationship and client collaboration: applying the Intentional Relationship model. In: Boyt Schell BA, Gillen G, eds. *Willard & Spackman's Occupational Therapy*. 13th ed. Wolters Kluwer; 2019:527–538.

Trede F, Higgs J. Collaborative decision making. In: Higgs J, Jones M, Loftus S, Christensen N, eds. *Clinical Reasoning in the Health Professions*. 3rd ed. Butterworth Heinemann; 2008:31–41.

Turpin M. Recovery of our phenomenological knowledge in occupational therapy. *Am J Occup Ther*. 2007 Jul-Aug;61(4):481–485. doi:10.5014/ajot.61.4.469

Turpin M, Copley J. Interactive reasoning. In: Boyt Schell BA, Schell J, eds. *Clinical and Professional Reasoning in Occupational Therapy*. 3rd ed. Wolters Kluwer; 2023.

Turpin M, Fitzgerald C, Copley J, Laracy S, Lewis B. Experiences of and support for the transition to practice of newly graduated occupational therapists undertaking a hospital graduate program. *Aust Occup Ther J*. 2021 Feb;68(1):12–20. doi:10.1111/1440-1630.12693

Turpin M, Higgs J. Clinical reasoning and EBP. In: Hoffman T, Bennett S, Bennett J, Del Mar C, eds. *Evidence-Based Practice Across the Health Professions*. 3rd ed. Churchill Livingstone; 2017:300–317.

Unsworth CA. Using a head-mounted video camera to explore current conceptualizations of clinical reasoning in occupational therapy. *Am J Occup Ther*. 2005 Jan-Feb;59(1):31–40. doi:10.5014/ajot.59.1.31

Williams L, Lawlis T. The sociology of allied health. In: Germov J, ed. *Second Opinion: An Introduction to Health Sociology*. 6th ed. Oxford University Press; 2019:541–568.

World Federation of Occupational Therapists. Minimum standards for the education of occupational therapists, 2016. https://www.wfot.org/resources/new-minimum-standards-for-the-education-of-occupational-therapists-2016-e-copy

CHAPTER 3

Occupational Performance Models and Occupational Adaptation

CHAPTER CONTENTS

Occupational Performance Model   40
Main Concepts and Definitions of Terms   40
Intervention   42
Historical Description of Model's
   Development   45
Summary   46
Memory Aid   47
Major Works   47

**Occupational Performance Model
(Australia)   47**
Main Concepts and Definitions of Terms   48
   Occupational Performance (Construct 1)   49
   The Internal Context (Constructs 2
      Through 5)   50
   *Occupational Role: Where the Internal
      and External Contexts Connect
      (Construct 2)   50*
   *Occupational Performance Areas
      (Construct 3)   52*
   *Occupational Performance Capacities
      (Construct 4)   53*

*Core Elements of Occupational Performance
   (Construct 5)   54*
   The External Context (Construct 6)   55
   Space and Time (Constructs 7 and 8)   56
Historical Description of the Model's
   Development   56
Summary   57
Memory Aid   58
Major Works   58

Occupational Adaptation Model   58
Main Concepts and Definitions of Terms   59
Historical Description of the Model's
   Development   62
Summary   62
Memory Aid   63
Major Works   63

Conclusion   64

References   64

The story of formal occupational therapy models essentially starts with *occupational performance models*. These models represent the occupational therapy perspective articulated most prominently in North America from the post–World War II period to the 1980s. While occupational therapy in English-speaking countries grew out of both British and North American movements, the way occupational therapy has been conceptualized in North America has had a widespread influence on its theory throughout the world. While occupational performance models were developed in various Western countries—an example is the Canadian Occupational Performance Model (Department of National Health and Welfare and Canadian Association of Occupational Therapists 1983)—we have selected two that demonstrate different aspects of this approach: the Occupational Performance Model, or OPM (Pedretti and Early 2001), which originated in the

United States; and the Occupational Performance Model (Australia), or OPM(A) (Chapparo and Ranka 1997; Chaparro et al. 2017), which comes from Australia.

The OPM illustrates the essence of occupational performance models since the 1970s, a decade steeped in the biomedical perspective dominant at the time and centered on remediation of the body. In contrast, the OPM(A) was developed 25 years after the original occupational performance models, at a time when the biopsychosocial perspective was gaining acceptance in health culture in Western countries. The OPM and OPM(A) demonstrate key performance components and performance areas of occupational performance models that can be seen in previous versions of other occupational therapy models. One of these is the Canadian Model of Occupational Performance and Engagement (CMOP-E), the precursor to the Canadian Model of Occupational Participation (CanMOP), which identified affective, cognitive, and physical aspects of the person (performance components in the OPM) and categorized occupation as self-care, productivity, and leisure (performance areas in the OPM). The OPM and OPM(A) also illustrate the perspective shift brought about through the conceptual progression from a biomedical to a biopsychosocial perspective in health.

In addition to discussing the OPM and OPM(A) in detail, this chapter also covers the Theory of Occupational Adaptation (OA), also referred to as the Occupational Adaptation Model (OAM), which, as the name suggests, focuses on occupational adaptation rather than occupational performance. This model was devised by Janette Schkade and Sally Schultz (Schkade and Schultz 1992; Schultz and Schkade 1992) and was recently reconceptualized by Lenin Grajo (2017). As we progress through this chapter, we will see that the language used in occupational therapy has moved away from this normative-body focus toward participation in everyday life.

Occupational Performance Model

In this section, the OPM, as articulated by Lorraine Williams Pedretti and colleagues in the various editions of her well-known occupational therapy textbook *Occupational Therapy: Practice Skills for Physical Dysfunction* (1981, 1985, 1990, 1996, 2001), is presented in detail in its final form (subsequent editions of that textbook are edited by Pendleton and Schultz-Krohn and no longer present the OPM, but instead, the various editions of the Occupational Therapy Practice Framework [OTPF]). We chose to start with the OPM because the concepts in that model were so central to occupational therapy for such a long time. Many of these concepts have remained important (particularly in physical rehabilitation) and knowledge of them may help explain many of the current debates in occupational therapy, such as whether occupational therapists should use methods other than occupation in their practice. Pedretti and Early's (2001) statement, "occupational performance terminology [used in the model] was defined and standardized in official documents of the AOTA" (p. 4), demonstrates that the OPM encapsulated the officially accepted view of the domain of concern of occupational therapy by the American Occupational Therapy Association at the time.

MAIN CONCEPTS AND DEFINITIONS OF TERMS

Lorraine Williams Pedretti is the author most closely associated with articulating the OPM. She did not claim to have authored this model but explained that some components of the model "have always been the core of OT" (Pedretti and Early 2001, p. 4) and that other details were added by committees and task forces of the AOTA during the 1970s. The diagram (1996, 2001) used to represent the model (see Fig. 3.1) acknowledges that it is based on the uniform terminology for occupational therapists, which was published in three editions by the AOTA and was succeeded by the OTPF (the fourth edition, OTPF-4, is presented in Chapter 5). Throughout the description of the OPM, the term *patient* is used, as that is the term most often used in relation to this

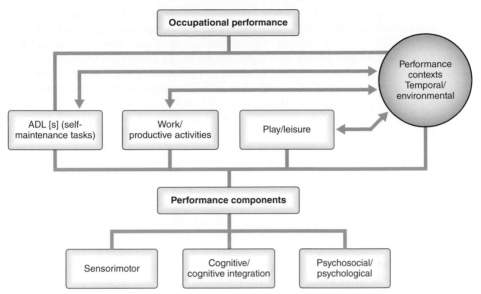

Fig. 3.1 Occupational Performance Model (as presented by Pedretti and Early 1996, 2001).

model. That is, the model used the term *patient* to refer to the subject of therapy, and for consistency, we do the same.

As the name suggests, the central aim in this model is to facilitate occupational performance. *Occupational performance* was defined as "the ability to perform those tasks that make it possible to carry out occupational roles in a satisfying manner appropriate for the individual's developmental stage, culture, and environment" (Pedretti and Early 2001, p. 5). Pedretti defined *occupational roles* as "the life roles that an individual holds in society" (1996, p. 3). Occupational roles develop in conjunction with the occupations in which people engage and include roles such as "pre-schooler, student, parent, homemaker, employee, volunteer, or retired worker" (2001, p. 5). Thus the purpose of occupational performance is to be able to fulfill occupational roles.

Facilitating occupational performance is dependent upon sufficient opportunities to practice and learn the skills and abilities required for occupational roles and developmental tasks. The OPM provides a framework for occupational therapists to systematically analyze the problems that are reducing the occupational performance of an individual. It comprises three elements: (1) performance areas (activities of daily living or ADLs, work/productive activities, and play/leisure); (2) performance components (sensorimotor, cognitive/cognitive integration, and psychosocial/psychological); and (3) performance contexts (temporal/environmental). Problems that interfere with occupational performance might stem from "deficits in task learning experiences, performance components, or impoverished performance contexts" (Pedretti and Early 2001, p. 5).

The *performance areas* are the first of the three elements described in the model. Activities are grouped into three performance areas: ADLs, work and productive activities, and play or leisure activities. As Pedretti and Early (2001) explained, "ADL[s] include the self-maintenance tasks of grooming, hygiene, dressing, feeding and eating, mobility, socialization, communication, and sexual expression. Work and productive activities include home management, care of others, educational activities, and vocational activities. Play and leisure include play exploration and play or leisure performance in age-appropriate activities." (p. 5.) The model places a primacy on the performance areas because of their vital contribution to occupational roles.

Performance components have been defined as "the learned developmental patterns of behavior which are the substructure and foundation of the individual's occupational performance" (Pedretti and Early 2001, p. 5). An understanding of performance components is based on developmental theory. As people grow, they develop these capacities. According to this model, "adequate neurophysiological development and integrated functioning of the performance components are basic to an individual's ability to perform occupational tasks or activities in the performance areas" (pp. 5–6). From this perspective, identification of people's capacities in terms of these components of performance can shed light on where occupational performance might be breaking down. Performance components are categorized into three groups: (1) sensorimotor, (2) cognitive and cognitive integration, and (3) psychosocial and psychological. The sensorimotor component includes sensory, neuromusculoskeletal, and motor functions. The cognitive and cognitive integration components relate to the ability to use higher brain functions. The psychosocial and psychological components include those abilities required for social interaction and emotional processing. The model provides substantial detail about the nature of these performance components (see Table 3.1). For several decades, occupational therapy in rehabilitation was highly focused on identification and remediation of problems with performance components. However, while a detailed understanding of performance components is essential, Pedretti and Early emphasized that "intervention strategies must ultimately be directed to the patient's achievement in performance areas when a performance component (e.g., motor skill development) is being addressed" (p. 6). We are reminded that, while the performance components provide details for occupational therapists that are particularly useful in planning rehabilitation interventions, occupational therapy intervention should always be aimed at promoting those components required for performance of a person's occupational roles.

The third element in the OPM is *performance contexts*. The model acknowledges that occupational performance is conducted in a variety of contexts that shape occupational demands. Performance contexts are conceptualized as temporal and environmental. Pedretti and Early (2001) listed as examples of the temporal context "the individual's age, developmental stage or phase of maturation, and stage in important life processes such as parenting, education, or career," and they emphasized that "disability status (e.g., acute, chronic, terminal, improving, or declining) must also be considered" (p. 6). These examples suggest that, in this model, the temporal contexts appear to relate primarily to the individual. Environmental dimensions of the performance contexts are considered under the categories of physical, social, and cultural. As Pedretti and Early stated, "The physical environment includes homes, buildings, outdoors, furniture, tools, and other objects. Social environment includes significant others and social groups. Cultural environment includes customs, beliefs, standards of behavior, political factors, and opportunities for education, employment, and economic support" (p. 6).

INTERVENTION

Underlying the model are two key approaches to facilitating occupational performance: remediation and compensation. In a *remediation* approach, intervention is targeted toward improving performance components, with the assumption that such improvements will lead to enhanced occupational performance in the performance areas. A *compensatory* approach is used when remediation is not considered achievable or feasible. According to Pedretti and Early (2001), the compensatory approach "focuses on remaining abilities and aims to improve function by adapting or compensating for performance component deficits" (p. 6). They proposed that examples of this approach might include adapting the methods used to perform tasks, providing assistive devices, or modifying the environment.

The OPM outlines four levels of intervention. Because remediation is the center of this model (essentially, remediation is the preferred approach and compensation is only used when remediation does not appear to be achievable or feasible), these four levels primarily categorize methods that could be used for the remediation of problems in performance components. The four levels, in

TABLE 3.1 ■ Performance Components of the OP Model

Sensory Functions	Sensorimotor Components / Neuromusculoskeletal Functions	Motor Functions	Cognitive Integration and Cognitive Components	Psychosocial and Psychological Components
• Sensory awareness and processing and perceptual processing	• Reflex responses • Range of motion • Musc e tone • Strength • Endurance • Postural control • Postural alignment • Soft-t ssue integrity	• Gross coordination • Crossing the midline • Laterality • Bilateral integration • Motor control • Praxis • Fine coordination and dexterity • Oral motor control	• Level of arousal • Orientation • Recognition • Attention span • Initiation of activity • Termination of activity • Memory • Sequencing • Categorization • Concept formation • Spatial operations • Problem solving • Learning • Generalization	• Values • Interests • Self-concept • Role performance • Social conduct • Interpersonal skills • Self-expression • Coping skills • Time management • Self-control

sequence, are (1) adjunctive methods, (2) enabling activities, (3) purposeful activity, and (4) occupations. Together, they represent an intervention continuum that "takes the patient through a logical progression from dependence to occupational performance to resumption of valued social and occupational roles" (Pedretti and Early 2001, p. 7). However, this continuum is not meant to be used in a strictly stepwise fashion, and the various levels can overlap and be used simultaneously as required. Essentially, these intervention levels are based on the premise that purposeful activity is the "primary treatment tool of occupational therapy" (p. 7) and that adjunctive methods and enabling activities are used as "preparatory" to functional activity in performance areas. The aim of remediating problems in the performance components is not an end in itself, and as the authors stated, "exclusive use of such preparatory methods out of context of the patient's occupational performance is not considered OT" (p. 7). The four levels are used in combination to promote participation in occupational roles.

The first level of intervention is *adjunctive methods*. These are "procedures that prepare the patient for occupational performance but are preliminary to the use of purposeful activity" (p. 7). These methods generally focus on remediating performance components or maintaining structural integrity of body parts to prevent problems that could interfere with their potential use. They include methods such as "exercise, facilitation and inhibition techniques, positioning, sensory stimulation, selected physical agent modalities, and provision of devices such as braces and splints" (p. 7). Pedretti and Early (2001) emphasized that occupational therapists using these methods need to plan for progression to the subsequent intervention levels to ensure that adjunctive methods remain preparatory to purposeful activity.

The second level is *enabling activities*. This level involves the use of activities that might not be considered purposeful. Interventions at this level often involve simulation tasks, examples of which include "sanding boards, skateboards, stacking cones or blocks, practice boards for mastery of clothing fasteners and hardware, driving simulators, work simulators, and tabletop activities such as form boards for training in perceptual-motor skills" (Pedretti and Early 2001, p. 7). These are often used when the requirements of purposeful activities are beyond the capabilities of patients. Essentially, they represent graded activities that might enable patients to engage in activities for remediation and experience success and are used when purposeful activities would not likely result in this level of success. However, like adjunct methods, they need to be regarded as preparatory to purposeful activity. The primary goal of the first two levels of intervention is the remediation of performance components.

Pedretti and Early (2001) also included the use of equipment in this second level. They listed equipment such as "wheelchairs, ambulatory aids, special clothing, communication devices, environmental control systems, and other assistive devices" (p. 7) as interventions at this level. This is consistent with the imperative that enabling activities should only be preparatory to purposeful activities. In the same way, devices and equipment should not be seen as ends in themselves, but as a means of enabling engagement in purposeful activities and occupation. They serve the purpose of enabling!

The third intervention level is *purposeful activity*. Pedretti and Early (2001) emphasized that purposeful activity has always been at the core of occupational therapy. They defined purposeful activities as "activities that have an inherent or autonomous goal and are relevant and meaningful to the patient" (p. 8). It is the goal, relevance, and meaningfulness to the patient that distinguishes this level from the second level, in which the activities chosen might have a goal that is meaningful to the occupational therapist but that might not be evident to or valued by the client. The model assumes that activities become meaningful and purposeful to an individual because they are required in that person's performance areas. Therefore it is their contribution to the performance areas that makes activities purposeful.

At this level of intervention, purposeful activity is used for "assessing and remediating deficits in the performance areas" (Pedretti and Early 2001, p. 8). Thus, in this third level, attention shifts to performance areas (compared with concentration on performance components at the first two levels). Examples of activities used are "feeding, hygiene, dressing, mobility, communication, arts, crafts, games, sports, work, and educational activities" (p. 8), and they could be conducted in the patient's home, a community agency, or a healthcare facility.

The final level of intervention refers to *occupations*. This is the highest point in the treatment continuum and involves engaging "the patient in natural occupations in his or her living environment and in the community. The patient performs appropriate tasks of ADL[s], work and productive activities, and play and leisure to his or her maximum level of independence." (p. 9.) Because the core of this level is maximum independence and these activities are performed in their natural environments, active involvement in "scheduled OT" (p. 9) decreases to the point where it terminates and the individual "resumes and effectively performs valued occupational roles" (p. 9). The focus of this level of intervention moves to the performance of occupational roles within their natural context, with occupational therapy intervention trailing off until it is no longer required.

Pedretti and Early (2001) identified two "intervention approaches" (p. 10) that are valuable to use in conjunction with the OPM in the practice area of physical dysfunction: the biomechanical model and the motor control model. Each approach provides principles for the treatment of movement problems caused by different processes.

The *biomechanical model* "applies the mechanical principles of kinetics and kinematics to the movement of the human body. These mechanical principles deal with the way that forces acting on the body affect movement and equilibrium." (p. 10.) The biomechanical model guides the assessment and restoration of range of motion, muscle strength and endurance (muscular and cardiovascular) and the prevention and reduction of deformity. The biomechanical model is used for individuals with sensorimotor problems resulting from "motor unit or orthopedic disorders but whose central nervous system (CNS) is intact" (p. 10). Common intervention methods include "joint measurement, muscle strength testing, kinetic activity, therapeutic exercise, and orthotics" (p. 10), and many of the common interventions from the first two levels—adjunctive methods and enabling activities—derive from the biomechanical model.

The *motor control model* addresses CNS problems. Pedretti and Early (2001) identified four approaches within this model: (1) the Rood approach to movement therapy; (2) the Brunnstrom approach to movement therapy; (3) Knott and Voss's proprioceptive neuromuscular facilitation; and (4) Bobath's neurodevelopmental treatment. More recent publications of texts on rehabilitation for CNS problems demonstrate that the specific models used for addressing these types of problems have changed as knowledge has developed in this area. Readers are referred to more recent publications for the current approaches in this area.

The biomechanical and motor control treatment approaches (often called *frames of reference* by other authors) are utilized in combination with the OPM to address problems in the sensorimotor performance components. Occupational therapists typically combine the OPM with other treatment approaches to provide details of interventions for other performance components. For example, they might use a cognitive behavioral approach to understand interventions for psychosocial problems.

HISTORICAL DESCRIPTION OF MODEL'S DEVELOPMENT

Despite the OPM being somewhat dated and no longer formally published, it is arguably the model that has influenced most pervasively the thinking of many practicing occupational therapists throughout the world. This applies particularly to the area of physical dysfunction (but originally more broadly).

The OPM reflected the official stance of the AOTA and was influenced by the documents the association produced from the early 1970s. In 1996, Pedretti provided a detailed description of the history of the development of the OPM. She commenced by stating:

> In 1973 the American Occupational Therapy Association (AOTA) published The Roles and Functions of Occupational Therapy Personnel. *This publication referred to occupational*

performance as a frame of reference that included three performance skills, later named perfor-
mance areas, and five performance components, later combined to become the three used in the
later versions of the [OPM]. The purpose was to describe the areas of expertise of occupational
therapists and the domains of concern within the profession. (p. 5.)

In this history, Pedretti discussed various publications created throughout the 1970s and early
1980s as contributing to an understanding of occupational performance. She also cited the three
editions of the AOTA publication outlining recommendations for uniform reporting of occupational therapy services (which were primarily centered on hospital-based services) as documents
that "defined the terminology in the occupational performance frame of reference" (p. 5). In
summarizing its development, she wrote:

Thus, the concept of the Occupational Performance model was developed from a series of task
forces and committees of the AOTA. It was generated from professional conceptualizations of
practice and originally described as a frame of reference for practice and for curriculum design
in education. (p. 5.)

The post–World War II period represents a major change in occupational therapy thinking in Western societies. Originally, the founders of occupational therapy conceptualized
occupation as treatment to engage people to become productive members of society and
focused on recreation, daily activities, and work (Hinojoa et al. 2017). However, as the social
context changed, so too did notions of occupation. While occupational therapy had commenced in mental health, the world wars led to an increase in physical rehabilitation with a
heightened medical focus. As Friedland (1998) explained, after WWII, occupational therapy's understanding of occupation as "a means of enhancing medical outcomes became firmly
established" (p. 377). According to Friedland, this biomedical perspective dominated occupational therapy thinking through the subsequent decades, "with periodic visits back to core
concepts" (p. 374) by authors such as Reilly (1962) and others. Occupational performance
models use the language of science, which also forms the basis of a biomedical (and biopsychosocial) perspective. This is evident in the two occupational performance models presented
in this chapter through their use of knowledge bases relating to the anatomy and physiology
of the body.

Evident within the OPM presented here is the influence of both mechanistic paradigm and
the beginning of a return to occupation (both of which are discussed in the introduction to this
book; see Table I.1). The OPM provides a structure that guides occupational therapists to analyze
performance components in detail and to use remediation and compensation to facilitate occupational performance. While providing guidance for rehabilitation conducted in biomedical
contexts, the model emphasizes that all treatment activities should be directed to the purpose of
facilitating the performance of occupational roles.

SUMMARY

The OPM demonstrates the major threads in occupational therapy thinking in the United
States in the post–World War II period. While the OPM has not been published in a substantial period of time, its legacy has remained in occupational therapy practice in Western countries. In Box 3.1 we present a memory aid for the OPM to help make explicit how it would be
used in practice. With the renaissance of occupation, the discourse of occupational therapy has
changed since the latter part of the 20th century and the term *occupation* is now used pervasively.
In the sections that follow, we can see this continuation of the renaissance of occupation in the
OPM(A) and the OAM.

MEMORY AID

See Box 3.1.

BOX 3.1 ■ OPM Memory Aid

Occupational Roles

What are the person's occupational roles?

For Each Role

- What purposes do they fulfill in the person's life?
- How does the person feel about these roles?
- How do these roles influence the person's self-identity and access to social and financial resources?

In which roles, if any, is the person likely to encounter problems with performance of those roles?

- Which roles are unlikely to be affected?

How is the context in which those roles are performed likely to affect, if at all, that performance?

Performance Areas

In the following areas, what activities does the person need/want to do to fulfill their occupational roles?

1. Activities of daily living (ADLs)
2. Work/productivity
3. Leisure/play

Performance Components

How is the person's capacities in the following areas influencing (if at all) their performance of the aforementioned activities and occupational roles?

1. Sensorimotor
2. Cognitive/cognitive integration
3. Psychosocial and psychological

MAJOR WORKS

Pedretti LW. Occupational performance: a model for practice in physical dysfunction. In: Pedretti LW, ed. *Occupational Therapy: Practice Skills for Physical Dysfunction*. 4th ed. Mosby; 1996:3–12.

Pedretti LW, Early MB. Occupational performance and models of practice for physical dysfunction. In: Pedretti LW, Early MB, eds. *Occupational Therapy: Practice Skills for Physical Dysfunction*. 5th ed. Mosby; 2001:3–12.

Occupational Performance Model (Australia)

Developed in 1997, the Occupational Performance Model (Australia), or OPM(A) (Chapparo and Ranka 1997; Chaparro et al. 2017) does not represent the official position of Occupational Therapy Australia (OTA) in the way the OPM represented the official position of the AOTA in the past. However, the OPM(A) provides an excellent example of an occupational performance model developed for a changed context in which the biopsychosocial model of health had become dominant. In addition to the biopsychosocial influences that are evident in the model, the philosophical basis of pragmatism that underpins the OPM(A) has more recently been made explicit (Chaparro et al. 2017). Pragmatism takes a holistic view of humans, rejecting any "dichotomies like mind-body, thought-action, rational-practical, and function-structure that presumed people could be divided into parts" (Hooper and Wood 2002, p. 41). Instead, it presents people as integrated, embodied beings that live and act in specific physical and social contexts that shape (afford and constrain) their actions toward their desired futures. Pragmatism emphasizes the primacy of a person's experiences and actions toward desired futures, which are always entwined with the specific physical and social contexts in which they occur. While the model incorporates traditional concepts from occupational performance models designed to break down performance into its elements, such as performance components, it emphasizes the holistic view of the person as an active agent embedded in context. Chapparo et al. (2017) stated that OPM(A) provides a framework for practice based of the following principles:

- "The perspectives, practices and outcomes of therapy are those that are *important to the person or group receiving occupational therapy.*
- The focus of therapy practice is on *real-world events* rather than artificial or manipulated scenarios." (p. 136, italics in original.)

Chaparro et al. (2017) emphasized that, while the OPM(A) takes a holistic view, this doesn't mean it uses generalizations. Instead, it rejects general notions such as *normative* and *typical* and attends to people and groups in their specificity (i.e., exactly as they *are*, rather than imposing any view of what they *should* be). Consequently, the model is concerned with the meanings people form regarding events, circumstances, and their own actions and those of others. Through attending to particularities with detail and nuance, the OPM(A) provides an excellent framework for analyzing the occupational performance of people and groups in their specific contexts at particular times. As Chaparro et al. (2017) stated, "the primary focus of the OPM(A) is the lifelong person–context relationship and its activation through occupation" (p. 136).

MAIN CONCEPTS AND DEFINITIONS OF TERMS

The OPM(A) is composed of eight constructs, which we will identify as we describe the model. As the name suggests, the OPM(A) focuses on occupational performance as its central concept (construct 1). It is concerned with specific people or groups performing occupation in specific contexts. The overall structure of the OPM(A) resonates with that of the OPM in that it outlines elements of occupational performance (the OPM has performance areas, performance components, and performance contexts). However, the OPM(A) differs from earlier occupational performance models by emphasizing that people are embedded in their context; this contrasts with Pedretti's model, in which the environment is depicted as a circle at the top right-hand corner of the model. It emphasizes this interconnectedness by using the language of *internal* and *external* contexts (i.e., contexts that are internal or external to the person, rather than identifying person and environment as separate entities). Fig. 3.2 provides a diagram of the OPM(A). It shows the internal context (i.e., internal to the person) comprising four elements, surrounded by the external context, with its seven elements.

Chaparro et al. (2017) further explained that the internal context is the core of the model. Its four elements are occupational role (construct 2), occupational performance areas (construct 3), occupational performance capacities (construct 4), and core elements of occupational performance (construct 5), and they are connected in the diagram by a complex array of lines. These four elements are embedded in the external context (construct 6), which includes psychological, cognitive, sensory, social, physical, cultural, spiritual, economic, and political aspects. Pervading this interconnected whole (internal and external contexts) are space (construct 7) and time (construct 8).

The features of the OPM(A) that distinguish it from earlier occupational performance models are consistent with other models developed or updated in the 1990s. These trends are toward (1) a more integrated view of the environment and its influence on occupational performance; (2) an increased focus on and use of the term *occupation* rather than *activity*; and (3) a biopsychosocial understanding of the person as consisting of subjective perceptions and experiences as well as body functions and structures. However, in a recent iteration (Chaparro et al. 2017), the model has moved beyond its original biopsychosocial understanding of the person to present the process of occupational performance as transactional, which is characteristic of a pragmatist perspective. This changed

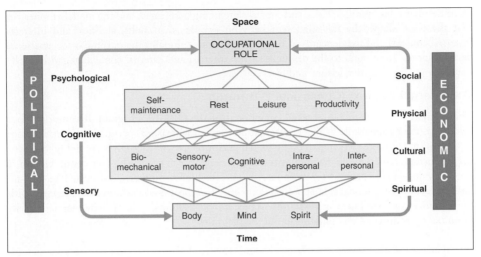

Fig. 3.2 Occupational Performance Model (Australia). (From Chapparo C, Ranka J, Nott M. Occupational Performance Model (Australia): a description of constructs, structure and propositions. In: Curtin M, Egan M, Adams J, eds. *Occupational Therapy for People Experiencing Illness, Injury or Impairment: Promoting Occupation and Participation.* 7th ed. Elsevier; 2017:136.)

understanding reflects the current times. For example, a transactional perspective is consistent with the dynamic biopsychosocial model of health proposed by Lehman et al. (2017), in which the bio-psychosocial model is reinterpreted within a dynamic systems perspective whereby an individual's health is directly shaped by context and historical time. A transactional perspective is particularly evident in the way the OPM(A) conceptualizes the internal context as comprising both the performer(s) and the occupation(s) being performed. Performer and occupation are not considered to exist separately, but occupation manifests only when it is performed and occupational performance is dependent on the congruence between a person's capacities and the demands of the occupation.

Having provided a background on the eight constructs, we will now discuss each construct in more detail.

Occupational Performance (Construct 1)

Occupational performance is the major focus of the OPM(A). While it is the primary construct, it pervades the entire model and does not appear as a separate concept in the OPM(A) diagram. Chapparo et al. (2017) defined it as "the ability to perceive, desire, recall, plan and carry out roles, routines, tasks and sub-tasks for the purpose of self-maintenance, productivity, leisure and rest in response to demands of the internal and/or external context" (p. 137).

This definition has three aspects: (1) the process involved, (2) what is being performed, and (3) the purpose of that performance. In terms of the process, occupational performance commences with perceiving and desiring. In any situation, people must first perceive the need for occupational performance and desire it. This points to the inclusion of and focus on people's subjective experiences, whereby occupational performance depends upon their perceptions and experiences of the world and their place within it. Their desire for occupational performance is often generated from their occupational roles and what they want and need to do to fulfill them. These specific occupational roles are shaped by both people's own agency and the demands of the external context. After perceiving and desiring, the process involves recalling, planning, and carrying out. People need to be able to recall what they have determined to be required for their occupational roles, plan for how these will be undertaken, and then carry them out. The definition identifies that roles, routines, tasks, and subtasks are being performed, and the model emphasizes that these are shaped by the alignment between people's own skills, abilities, and interests (internal context) and the demands of the external context. Finally, the purpose of occupational performance is to respond to the demands of the internal and external contexts regarding self-maintenance, productivity, leisure, and rest.

The Internal Context (Constructs 2 Through 5)

The internal context forms the central component of the OPM(A) diagram. It comprises four levels: (1) occupational roles, (2) occupational performance areas, (3) occupational performance capacities, and (4) core elements of occupational performance. All four levels are richly interconnected, as represented in the diagram by multiple lines between the levels. This connectedness is also evident in each construct's definitions, which often refer to other constructs. The top and bottom levels, occupational role and core elements of occupational performance, intersect with the external context. The particular importance of occupational role is demonstrated by its prominent position and its capitalization in the diagram.

Occupational Role: Where the Internal and External Contexts Connect (Construct 2). Occupational role is the principal organizing feature of everyday life. Chaparro et al. (2017) defined occupational role as:

> *patterns of occupational behaviour composed of configurations of self-maintenance, productivity, leisure/play and rest occupations. Occupational roles are determined by each unique person-context-performance relationship. They are established through need and/or choice and are modified with age, ability, experience, circumstance and time. (p. 137, italics in original.)*

This definition demonstrates the way occupational role is richly intertwined with other components of the model. It forms both the apex of the internal context and the connection between the internal and external contexts. Because of this connection, occupational roles have implications for both self-identity and social participation. It is through action that people develop a sense of themselves and their place in the world.

Individuals have unique constellations of roles that create specific demands for occupational performance, depending upon their life circumstances, goals, and desires. At any one time, individuals hold a multitude of interconnecting roles. For example, they might simultaneously be a friend, family member, worker, service user, club member, and so forth. Associated with each role is a range of tasks, and the way each role needs to be approached and performed is dependent on context. For example, performing a role in a familiar environment is much more likely to be automatic than when undertaken in a new environment; in the role of worker, changing jobs will require a new range of tasks. The importance of each occupational role will vary among different people. As Chaparro et al. (2017) explained, "premium value may be assigned to any of these roles. For example, a person might value the role of friend over other interlocking roles at work" (p. 137). Some roles will be more important to a person because they are self-defining or because they are required by circumstances, while the performance of other roles might not matter to them. Over the course of an ordinary day, people will transition between their multiple roles. Often, this will occur quite seamlessly, without the transition being noticed. But sometimes people have difficulty transitioning between roles, perhaps because they are not sure which role is most appropriate for the circumstance. Because occupational roles lie at the interface between the internal and external contexts, they influence and are influenced by both. For example, the external context will affect the degree of choice an individual has over their occupational roles, and an individual will take on and carry out occupational roles according to their interests, capabilities, needs, and aspirations.

Role change is a feature of life. The OPM(A) definition of *occupational role* makes it clear that role configurations alter with "*age, ability, experience, circumstance* and *time*" (Chapparo et al. 2017, p. 137). While a person generally fulfills multiple roles simultaneously, these roles and their combinations will change as the internal and external contexts change. Internal contexts vary as people age; their capacities, skills, and interests wax and wane; and their experiences and expectations of and hopes for life change. Over the course of a person's life, roles can be lost and gained and may be altered at different times. For example, the role of parent will change as a person's child grows up. What people do and the roles they hold when they are children and when they are adults will vary. Similarly, younger adults' roles differ from those of older adults. Often, acquiring a disability can result in the loss of some roles and the gain of others. The gaining and relinquishing of roles may be temporary, longer term, or permanent and may result from personal choice or be imposed. External contexts also contribute to role change as other people come and go; the physical contexts in which people perform occupational roles are altered and vary; and societies, organizations, and institutions change. As the internal and external contexts change, the demands placed on people combine with their preferences, abilities, and perceptions of choice to influence their roles and the performance of those roles.

The occupational roles of any specific person are configured uniquely according to the distinctive *person-context-performance relationship*. That is, occupational roles depend on both the person's own interpretation of what is required and the expectations of others (of both society generally and of significant individuals), as well as on the demands of the tasks being performed in the relevant context. Rather than individuals making unilateral decisions about their occupational roles, the interaction between the internal and external contexts shapes determination of these roles. Expectations about role performance arise from a combination of sociocultural factors in the external environment and those internal to the person performing the role (both personal preferences and beliefs and values internalized from the external environment throughout their life course). Thus society places expectations on how certain roles should be fulfilled, and each person brings their own unique skills and perspectives to performing that role, as well as their beliefs about what society expects of them in that role. How an individual undertakes a specific role will also depend on their perceptions of the value of that role in their life and what needs to be done to fulfill it. Thus the OPM(A) emphasizes the mutual influence of social and individual expectations and interpretations.

The result of this interplay will manifest differently in different societies. For example, some societies may emphasize personal choice while the notion of individual choice may be an anathema in more collectivist societies. Chapparo et al. (2017) explained that the relationship between the implications of personal choices and the demand of the sociocultural context is complex. Over time, people generally create a balance in their lives between what others expect and demand of them and their own personal desires. However, this balance can be disrupted with the onset of health problems and consequent alterations in personal capacities and by changed demands from the context.

Occupational roles can fulfill different purposes in people's lives and can influence their perceptions of themselves as well is the capacities and skills they develop. The position of occupational roles at the intersection of internal and external contexts emphasizes that both influence choices and perceptions of need, shaping the purposes they fulfill in each person's life. For example, a person might perceive the need to engage in a particular occupational role in a particular way to address a social demand. However, fulfilling this role might also affect how that person thinks about themselves (self-identity) and might influence the capacities, skills, and interests they develop (the external context shapes self-identity and capacity development). If a person's role performance is evaluated positively by both the external and internal contexts (i.e., others and themselves), that person is likely to enjoy and pursue that role and it might become increasingly self-defining. In contrast, if they feel they have no choice but to perform that role, they might see it as a duty or as essential for survival (or some other social purpose) rather than something to look forward to. However, it might still be self-defining if they take pride in performing the role well.

How people approach an occupational role will depend on the feedback obtained from the external context as well as their own interpretation of the situation, which always depends on a person's internalized sociocultural views.

Drawing on a pragmatist perspective, Chapparo et al. (2017) proposed that occupational roles have three mutually influencing dimensions: knowing, doing, and being. These contribute to occupational role performance to different degrees, depending on the abilities of the person and the demands of the role. *Knowing* involves "having an intuitive or concrete understanding of the roles people want to enact and what roles are expected by their physical-sensory-sociocultural context" (p. 138). In a sense, it is about identifying valued roles (the impetus for value being both internal and external) and knowing what each requires. The *doing* element refers to the process of carrying out occupational performance roles. Thus it is not enough just to know what is required. One also needs to be able to *do* what is required. While this generally relates to people's own performance, it may also include the action of instructing others to carry out or perform occupations on their behalf. Finally, occupational roles have interpersonal and socioemotional implications for role identity. The fulfillment and satisfaction people gain from their occupational roles shape their sense of self: their *being*.

In illustrating these three dimensions, Chapparo et al. (2017) explained that people can fully or partially participate in occupational role performance. They gave the example of a homemaker who knows what the family needs (*knowing*), performs many tasks and routines (*doing*), and feels competent and perceives the role as having sociocultural value, thereby gaining fulfillment and satisfaction from the role (*being*). In contrast, an elderly person who needs considerable assistance in self-care tasks might only partially participate in the occupational role as self-maintainer. They might know what they want done (*knowing*) and instruct others on how to perform the task (*doing*), thus feeling satisfied with this aspect of their life (*being*). Another person might be unable to contribute to both the knowing and doing aspects of an occupational role, and their family might take responsibility for ensuring that they are well cared for. In this way, their sense of *being* a family member is confirmed.

Occupational Performance Areas (Construct 3)
This level is directly connected to occupational roles. There are four occupational performance areas: *self-maintenance, productivity, leisure/play,* and *rest* occupations. As Chapparo et al. (2017) explained, occupational therapy has traditionally categorized occupational performance into the three areas of *self-maintenance, productivity/school occupations,* and *leisure/play.* The OPM(A) adds *rest* as a fourth occupational performance area, as follows:

> **Rest occupations** *are defined as "the* purposeful pursuit *of* nonactivity. *This can include time devoted to* sleep *as well as routines, tasks, subtasks and rituals undertaken in order to* relax" *(Chapparo et al. 2017, p, 139).*

This occupational performance area was included because of the many reasons related to lifespan, daily life, and sociocultural factors that might cause people to want to be still and quiet rather than active. This rationale acknowledges that the external context influences a person's occupational behavior. Whereas categorizing rest as self-maintenance would emphasize its role in the moderation of the internal environment, keeping it separate allows space for including the need or choice to respond to external demands and influences. For example, resting and relaxing through nonactivity can have a social purpose.

The remaining three occupational performance areas are defined as follows:

> **Self-maintenance occupations** *are routines, tasks, and subtasks done to* preserve *a person's* health *and* well-being *in the environment (Reed 2005). These routines, tasks, and subtasks can be*

in the form of habitual routines (dressing, eating) or occasional nonhabitual tasks (taking medication for an acute condition) that are demanded by circumstance (Chapparo and Ranka 1997).

Productivity/school occupations *are routines, tasks, and subtasks done to enable a person to* engage in *learning and* provide support *for* self, family, *or* community *through the production of* goods *or provision of* services *(Chapparo and Ranka 1997; Reed 2005).*

Leisure/play occupations *are routines, tasks, and subtasks done for purposes of* attainment, creativity, *and* celebration *(Chapparo and Ranka 1997).*

Within the broad areas into which occupational performance can be categorized, the OPM(A) also identifies three units of performance. Commencing with the simplest and increasing in complexity, these are subtasks, tasks, and routines. Using the examples of drinking and eating, Chapparo et al. (2017) explained the three. *Subtasks* are observable behaviors that constitute "steps or single units" of tasks, such as reaching for a glass or spoon. *Tasks* are sequences of subtasks that are undertaken to achieve a certain purpose, can involve doing and/or planning, and have a specific beginning and end, such as grasping a drinking vessel, bringing it to one's lips, drinking, returning it to the table, and releasing it. *Routines* are purposefully sequenced tasks, such as all the tasks that are integrated into the routine of preparing and eating a meal. Routines can vary in terms of both structure and timing. First, their structure can be fixed or flexible. *Fixed structures* determine how a routine needs to be done, allowing little deviation in established sequences of tasks. For example, the nature of the physical context often determines the demands and sequence of the tasks involved. In contrast, *flexible structures* enable routines to be undertaken in a variety of ways. Chapparo et al. emphasized that the way they are done should be acceptable to both the performer and others. Second, the timing of routines can be regular (e.g., daily, weekly) or intermittent. Regular routines can often become habitual because regular practice enables the task to be performed without thinking. In contrast, intermittent routines are not carried out with consistency and therefore require higher levels of conscious attention because they prevent the development of habits. The temporal aspects of routines, tasks, and subtasks also vary with age, circumstance, and ability, and their importance is not determined by whether they are regular or intermittent.

Chapparo et al. (2017) stressed that classifying tasks and routines into occupational performance areas is an idiosyncratic process. Tasks and routines do not have inherent meaning; rather, meaning is determined by the performer. How specific people classify an occupation can change over their life course and from day to day, depending upon its purpose. For example, the task of reading could be work, leisure, self-maintenance, or rest, depending on its purpose. While classification into occupational performance areas is idiosyncratic, it is not solely an individual pursuit.

Because occupational performance is inherently contextual, sociocultural contexts will shape how people categorize their tasks and routines. However, the OPM(A) emphasizes that neither the value placed on occupational performance areas nor expectations regarding the amount of time spent in each occupational performance area should be imposed from the outside. For example, while work is generally valued more highly than leisure in industrialized societies (sociocultural context), what is important to each person should be determined. In addition, there are no internal divisions among the four occupational performance areas in the OPM(A) diagram. This emphasizes that categorization into these different areas is an internal and fluid process.

Occupational Performance Capacities (Construct 4). The next level of the internal context is occupational performance capacities. In the diagram, this level is shown below the occupational performance level, and these two levels are connected by multiple lines. While previous occupational performance models conceptualized this level as pertaining to the capacities of the performer, the OPM(A) presents occupational performance as dependent on the *fit* between the capacities of the performer and the demands of the occupations being performed in a particular context. By juxtaposing the capacities of the performer and the demands of the occupation, the fit (or lack thereof) between them becomes obvious. Because a person's capacities are always considered in relation to the demands of specific occupations (which, by definition, are important to occupational role performance), the OPM(A) avoids the pitfall for which the occupational performance models are generally criticized: focusing on and remediating a person's capacities in a normative, restorative way. The criticism usually laid is that such remediation is too far removed from occupation and too easily becomes an end in itself. In the OPM(A), a person's capacities are always considered in terms of the tasks they need to perform in their occupational roles.

As Chapparo et al. (2017) stated, "there are motor, sensory, cognitive and psychosocial dimensions to any task performed that prompt a person to use motor, sensory, cognitive, interpersonal and intrapersonal capacities in a particular or *strategic* manner" (p. 141). As with occupational performance areas, there are no lines in the diagram between the performance capacities to indicate that they influence one another. Five areas of performance capacities are identified, and each is presented from the perspective of the performer and the task being performed (Chapparo et al. 2017, p. 141).

Motor capacity (move): For the performer, this refers to "the operation and interaction of and between *physical structures* of the body during task performance. This can include range of motion, muscle strength, grasp, muscular and cardiovascular endurance, circulation, elimination of body waste, regulation of muscle activity, generation of motor responses and coordination." Regarding the task, it "refers to the physical attributes of the task, such as size, load, dimension and location of objects."

Sensory capacity (sense): This "refers to the registration of sensory stimuli and discrimination" required by the performer and the sensory aspects of the task "such as colour, texture, temperature, weight, movement, sound, smell and taste."

Cognitive capacity (think): This is the "operation and interaction of and between mental processes used [by the performer] during task performance. This can include thinking, perceiving, recognising, remembering, judging, learning, knowing, attending and problem-solving." It also refers to the cognitive dimensions of the task, which are determined by its symbolic and operational complexity.

Intrapersonal capacity (feel): This refers to the internal psychological processes used by the performer when performing the task. It can include "feelings, emotions, self-esteem, mood, affect, rationality and defense mechanisms." It includes the intrapersonal attributes stimulated by and required for performance of the task, including valuing, satisfaction, and motivation.

Interpersonal capacity (communicate): This refers to interaction with others when performing the task and can include "sharing, cooperation, empathy, verbal and non-verbal communication." It also includes the interpersonal demands of the task.

Core Elements of Occupational Performance (Construct 5). The last level of the internal context consists of the core elements of occupational performance, which are body, mind, and spirit. Chapparo et al. (2017) explained that, while each of these core elements is defined separately, they cannot function separately or be understood independently; rather, together they form a holistic view of people. They stated that this "reflects pragmatist views of an integrated being whose mind, body and soul seek harmony" (p. 142). They defined each as follows (pp. 142–143):

The **body element** refers to all the "tangible *physical* elements of human structure".

The **mind element** is "the core of a person's conscious and unconscious intellect that forms the basis of the person's ability to understand and reason".

The **spirit element** "is defined loosely as an aspect of humans that *seeks* a sense of *harmony* within self and between self, nature, others and in some cases an ultimate other; *seeks* an *existing mystery* to live; *inner conviction*; *hope* and *meaning*".

Chapparo and Ranka (1997) summed up the relationship between these different core elements of occupational performance by stating:

> *Together the body, mind, and spirit form the human body, the human brain, the human mind, the human consciousness of self and the human awareness of the universe. Relative to occupational performance, the body-mind-spirit core element of this model translates into the "doing-knowing-being" dimensions of performance. These doing-knowing-being dimensions are fundamental to all occupational roles, routines, tasks and subtasks and components of occupational performance. (p. 13.)*

These core elements present people as embodied beings who plan their actions according to the meaning they create in their lives.

The External Context (Construct 6)

Surrounding the four levels of the internal context is the external context. In the OPM(A) the external context is presented as "an interactive world which has physical, sensory, cognitive, psychological, social, cultural, spiritual, and political-economic elements" (Chapparo et al. 2017, p. 143). When people undertake occupational performance, they do it in specific contexts, which provide opportunities for and make demands on occupational performance. Thus the external context can facilitate or produce barriers to performing occupations. Chapparo et al. (2017, p. 144) explained each as follows:

> The **physical context** is "the physical, tangible elements of situations in which people perform or participate, the location and arrangement of objects in the physical world and the physical characteristics of tools, objects, equipment, materials, supplies, food and liquids used (e.g., size, dimension, position, weight, viscosity). This includes naturally occurring characteristics and those that are built, engineered, manufactured or assembled."

The **sensory context** refers to the sensory characteristics of everything used and includes "temperature, texture, sound, light, odour, taste, humidity, movement and vibration".

The **cognitive context** refers to the "cognitive and perceptual complexity of situations" in which occupational performance is undertaken as well as the ease with which information can be interpreted "in order to know what things are, what to do and how to use items." The cognitive context can include a virtual context.

The **psychological context** is defined as "the characteristics of situations that support or challenge a person's psyche. This includes dimensions that may invoke high levels of arousal, strong emotions, stress responses or have a calming effect."

The **social context** includes expectations of and demands for social interaction.

The **cultural context** refers to traditions and expectations transmitted from generation to generation. "These include cultural symbols, arrangement of space, tools and materials used, modes of dress, modes of interaction, place for rituals, customs and ceremonies."

The **spiritual context** comprises situations that support people's spiritual beliefs such as "places of worship and sacred sites or places to be meditative, [and] tools, materials, clothing and food associated with sacred rights and rituals."

The **political context** includes "the explicit and implicit laws, policies and rules that govern and regulate performance and participation".

The **economic context** is defined as "the explicit and implicit and financial systems and structures that fund and reward performance and participation".

This detailed understanding emphasizes the complexity of the contexts in which occupation is performed. Each element uniquely shapes occupational performance. Some aspects of the context make it easy for a particular person to undertake an occupation if the demands of the context match the person's capacities. If the fit is poor, occupational performance will be hindered. Contexts change constantly. For example, the contexts themselves might alter or people might move to a new context. Similarly, the tasks being undertaken will vary, with some tasks being easier to perform with certain contextual features than with others.

Space and Time (Constructs 7 and 8)

In the OPM(A), pervading occupational performance is the concept of *space*, which is defined as "an expanse that extends in all directions, in which all material objects or forms are located". In the OPM(A), space is presented in terms of physical space and felt space, which equate to the external and internal environments, respectively. The concept of *physical space* is based on physics and includes physical matter such as objects, body structures, and the wider physical world. *Felt space* refers to people's experience of the physical space surrounding them and their interpretation of that space. The model emphasizes that the way physical space is experienced (felt) during occupational performance pervades all levels of the internal context. For example, the size and shape of physical objects will activate receptors and responses at the performance capacity level and be interpreted at the level of the body-mind-spirit core elements, and this subjective experience will contribute to the performance of occupations and occupational roles.

As with space, *time* has external and internal dimensions. *Physical time* can be seen in processes like the measurement of time and the regular movement of the sun and moon. It underpins concepts like sequence and simultaneous occurrence. *Felt time* refers to a person's experience of time, which will vary according to circumstances and the tasks being completed. For example, if a person perceives they do not have time to carry out a task, time will feel pressured. In contrast, time will seem to stretch when there are no deadlines. Chapparo et al. (2017) gave examples of influences of time on occupational performance, such as the time taken for muscle contraction, sequential ordering of steps in a task, and tasks in a routine; the use of strategies when they are required; and being in the right place at the right time. Felt time is unique to individuals and varies among cultures.

HISTORICAL DESCRIPTION OF THE MODEL'S DEVELOPMENT

As with many of the practice models reviewed later in this book, the impetus for the development of the OPM(A) came from the need for a theoretical framework to guide the curriculum at a particular institution that trained occupational therapists. In this case it was the University of Sydney, in Australia. The authors stated that development of the model was commenced in 1986 "when it became clear that existing notions of occupational performance used to structure curriculum content in the Bachelor of Applied Science in Occupational Therapy at Cumberland College of Health Sciences (now The University of Sydney) required expansion to more adequately reflect both the nature of human occupations and occupational therapy practice" (Chapparo and Ranka 1997, p. 1).

Chapparo and Ranka (1997) explained that this school of occupational therapy was required to undergo curriculum reviews every five years and that, from the mid-1970s to the mid-1990s, the curriculum had changed considerably. They explained that the changes in this period led to "the development of a theoretical framework for the curriculum which [had] two integrated conceptual thrusts" (p. 24): (1) a movement toward "problem-based, adult learning modes of education"; and (2) the use of the "conceptual notions of occupational performance and functions to organize content within the curriculum" (p. 24).

As Chapparo and Ranka stated, "the process of model building was initially stimulated by curriculum restructuring and subsequently continued by the authors to develop a model of occupational performance that was relevant to occupational therapy practice in Australia" (p. 24).

They also stated that, in 1997, the OPM(A) was at the stage of development where "concepts have been developed, classified and related, but not yet fully evaluated or tested" (p. 2).

The model was developed in five stages:

Stage 1. 1989–1990: A review of the literature. This process led to the development of a model centered on occupational performance with two levels (presumably occupational performance areas and occupational performance components).

Stage 2. 1990–1991: "Field testing" (p. 28) of this model in the practice areas of neurology and adult rehabilitation. This led to the addition of a third level to the model (presumably occupational roles). The authors also added the construct of occupational performance environment, most likely conceptualized as surrounding the three levels in the model.

Stage 3. 1991–1992: Field testing the three-level model in acute care, pediatrics, and adult rehabilitation. This stage led to the addition of the fourth level of the model, which appears to have been the core elements of body, mind, and spirit. The authors also listed "development of philosophy and assumptions" (p. 28) as an outcome of this stage.

Stage 4. 1992–1994: Field testing the four-level model with the six constructs of (1) occupational performance, (2) occupational performance areas, (3) occupational performance components, (4) occupational roles, (5) occupational performance environment, and (6) core elements. This field testing was undertaken in the practice areas of adult rehabilitation, community pediatric practice, psychiatry, and occupational therapy administration. This stage led to acceptance of the four-level model with the addition of two further constructs: space and time.

Stage 5. 1994–1996: The final stage was described as "ongoing field testing" (p. 28) in which the constructs were consolidated and refined in practice contexts through the use of written examples provided to occupational therapists. The methods used in the field-testing stages of model development included continuing professional education workshops, and the use of "intervention scenarios" (p. 34) in which videotapes of clients and case studies were used as the stimulus for practitioners to plan interventions and discuss use in their own practice. Specific tasks were used to elicit practitioners' beliefs "about human potential, health, occupations, and occupational therapy" (p. 35) when developing a "personal frame of reference for practice" (p. 35).

Since the monograph was published in 1997, the model has been made available through its website (http://www.occupationalperformance.com) and Chaparro et al. (2017). One major change that occurred in the 2017 publication was use of the word *context* rather than *environment*. Chaparro et al. (2017) explained that the word *context* helps emphasize the difference between environments, which can have meanings that are shared by all, and the individual meanings people ascribe to the contexts in which they perform occupation. Several assessments have also been devised based on the OPM(A). These include the Perceive, Recall, Plan, and Perform (PRPP) system of task analysis and the Comparative Analyses of Performance (CAPs) (Chaparro and Ranka 1996).

SUMMARY

The OPM(A) provides an excellent demonstration of the trends that have occurred and are occurring in occupational therapy. When compared with the OPM, the OPM(A) demonstrates the difference in health between a biomedical and a biopsychosocial understanding of health and well-being. Often, this is described as the difference between a normative focus on rehabilitating the body and a focus on the whole person. However, the OPM(A) also foreshadows a more recent trend in occupational therapy that moves away from conceptualizing person, environment, and occupation as separate entities and toward a transactional whole. What would have been referred to at the time as *person* and *environment* are now referred to as *internal* and *external environments*, and occupation is the purpose of the model rather than a component of it. More recently, Chapparo et al. (2017) have linked this concept of a deeply transactional whole to the philosophy of pragmatism. Readers will see the transactional perspective feature in several chapters later in this book.

MEMORY AID

See Box 3.2.

BOX 3.2 ■ OPM(A) Memory Aid

What occupational roles does the person want or need to do?

For Each Role

- Which occupational performance area would the person use to categorize that role?
- What routines, tasks, and subtasks are needed for that person to fulfill that role?
- What occupational performance capacities (both the person's capacities and the activity demands) are required for performance of these routines, tasks, and subtasks?
- How are the body, mind, and spirit influencing and being influenced by role performance?
- How will the psychological, cognitive, sensory, social, physical, cultural, and spiritual environments influence and be influenced by performance of that role?
- How are space and time contributing to role performance?

MAJOR WORKS

Chapparo C, Ranka J. *OPM: Occupational Performance Model (Australia), Monograph 1*. Occupational Performance Network; 1997.

Chapparo C, Ranka J, Nott M. Occupational Performance Model (Australia): a description of constructs, structure and propositions. In: Curtin M, Egan M, Adams J, eds. *Occupational Therapy for People Experiencing Illness, Injury or Impairment: Promoting Occupation and Participation*. 7th ed. Elsevier; 2017:134–147.

Occupational Performance Model (Australia) website: http://www.occupationalperformance.com.

Occupational Adaptation Model

The third perspective presented in this chapter is the Theory of Occupational Adaptation (OA) (first published in two journal articles: Schkade and Schultz 1992; and Schultz and Schkade 1992). The terminology used to refer to OA has varied at different times. According to Schultz (2009), OA was introduced as a frame of reference in 1992, and in 2003 as an "overarching theory for occupational therapy practice and research" (p. 463). It was also referred to by Grajo as a model in 2017 and as a theory in 2019. OA differs from the OPM and OPM(A) in that they focus on occupational performance and OA centers on occupational adaptation. OA distinguishes between these two concepts by presenting occupational performance as a behavioral outcome and occupational adaptation as an internal process.

In reconceptualizing the process of occupational adaptation, Grajo (2019) explained that it "is a product of engagement and participation in occupations; a transaction with the environment; a manner of responding to change, altered situations, and life transitions; and a manner of forming identity" (p. 634). Grajo presented OA as both a normative, internal process and an intervention process. While Grajo (2017; 2019) has remained faithful to the essence of OA, one major change was the development a new diagram of the occupational adaptation process. As Grajo (2017) stated, the new diagram aimed "to highlight the multidimensional transactional event that occurs between the person and the environment rather than just a 'freeze frame' illustration" (p. 291); Schkade and Schultz (2003) had referred to their diagram as a "freeze-frame sketch" (p. 183) of the process of occupational adaptation. In this section, to offer a broad perspective of OA we draw upon a range of publications by the original authors, Janette Schkade and Sally Schultz, as well as those by Lenin Grajo.

MAIN CONCEPTS AND DEFINITIONS OF TERMS

OA aims to provide a theoretical framework for conceptualizing the process by which humans respond adaptively to their environments. The name "OA" comes from combining the concepts of occupation and adaptation, both foundational concepts for occupational therapy. A core assumption of occupational therapy is that occupation can be used to facilitate adaptation.

The main concern of OA is how people adapt to their environments through occupation. Central to OA is the principle that occupational adaptation is an internal process, which means it is a normal human process that occurs across the lifespan, rather than something that only occurs when illness, stress, or disability requires adaptation. As people grow and change, they need to continually adapt their responses to the environment. Emphasizing the normative concepts of adaptation, many publications encourage readers to apply OA to their own lives. For example, Schkade and McClung (2001) stated that, to enhance understanding of OA, "we recommend that a therapist wishing to use this perspective in intervention should first 'try it on' with regard to his or her own life role adaptation challenges" (pp. 2–3).

The quality of adaptation is presented in terms of *mastery*. Schkade and Schultz (2003) referred to mastery as a constant factor which is seen to manifest in three ways: (1) individuals *desire* mastery, (2) occupational environments *demand* it, and (3) their transaction *presses* for it. This combination of ideas about mastery is embedded within the diagrammatic representation of OA reconceptualized by Grajo (2019; see Fig. 3.3). At the bottom left of the diagram, the person is conceptualized as an occupational being with a desire for mastery. As Grajo (2017) explained, "the assertion by Mary Reilly (1962) that people are born with a desire to master and alter the environment is an important influence in the development of occupational adaptation" (p. 292). The innate nature of this need is central to OA (Schkade and McClung 2001; Schkade and Schultz 1992, 2003; Schultz 2009). People are motivated toward occupational engagement and participation by the desire for mastery.

At the top right of the diagram, occupational environment is understood as creating a demand for mastery from the person. As Schultz (2009) stated, "OA theory proposes that any circumstance presents itself with at least a minimal degree of demand for mastery" (p. 465). These demands can enable or restrict people's participation in occupation. The occupational environment includes physical, social, temporal, cultural, and virtual contexts. The various contexts in which people live place demands on them for action in terms of behavior, performance, and participation.

When people and occupational environments transact, they shape and change each other. As people engage in occupations, they impact on and change their environments. Similarly, the occupational environment's demands for mastery will shape how people respond and adapt. In OA, the person is conceptualized as consisting of unique sensorimotor, cognitive, and psychosocial systems, which are affected by biological, genetic, and phenomenological influences, all of which are required for occupation. Together, these three systems are referred to as the *Adaptation Gestalt*. The contributions of each system in the person's Adaptation Gestalt will vary according to the occupational environment. At times, the occupational environment might demand equal contributions of cognitive, sensorimotor, and psychosocial faculties. In other situations, more might be required of some systems than of others for a person to participate in occupation with mastery and competence.

In the center of the diagram are five cog shapes representing the components of the press for mastery. The press for mastery forms the centermost cog and is connected to the other four: occupational roles, occupational role demands, occupational challenges, and occupational

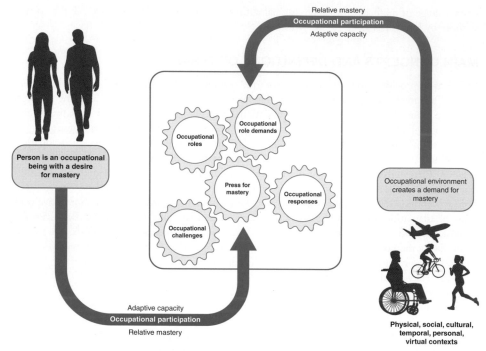

Fig. 3.3   Occupational Adaptation Model.

responses. As Grajo (2017) explained, "The press for mastery forms roles and role expectations that people need to fulfill, challenges that people need to conquer, and people's need to formulate a variety of responses to master the environment. Role expectations are central to the occupational adaptation process. Fulfillment of occupational roles and role expectations are important for people. Occupational roles create within people a sense of mastery and competence" (p. 296). The arrows in the diagram show that the transaction of person and occupational environment creates a press for mastery. It is this combination of desire, demand, and press for mastery that provides the impetus for humans to face occupational challenges and make adaptive responses. Adaptive responses are achieved through engagement in occupation, which is often demanded by roles. Earlier, Schultz (2009) explained the process in this way: "The *occupational role expectations* of the person and of the occupational environment intersect in response to the unique occupational challenge that the individual experiences. A demand for adaptation occurs. The person makes an internal adaptive response to the situation and then produces an *occupational response*. The *occupational response* is the outcome – the observable by-product of the adaptive response." (p. 465, italics in original.) The occupational response might be an action or a behavior. Overall, the process of occupational adaptation operates rapidly and repeatedly as people usually deal with multiple occupational challenges simultaneously.

Considering the process of responding to an occupational challenge, OA outlines the process by which people first prepare for and then carry out adaptive responses. When preparing to make a response, people use *adaptation energy*. For example, they might think directly about a problem, or they might think about it while doing something else. Either way, they are investing energy into formulating an adaptive response. They will also need to choose "adaptive patterns or strategies that [they have] established through life experiences" (Schultz 2009, p. 467). These could be new strategies, existing strategies, or modifications of existing strategies. Then, once they have used these three elements to prepare for generating a response, people gather their unique sensorimotor, cognitive, and psychosocial capacities, that is, their Adaptation Gestalt, and make the response.

Schultz (2009) clarified that individuals "produce an internal adaptive response to the occupational challenge" (p. 467) and that the occupational response is the product of this internal response. She went on to explain that "Although the adaptive response is not directly observable, it does become operationalized within the occupational response. The nature of the internal adaptive response can be gleaned readily from careful observation and analysis of the individual's approach to the task, his or her problem-solving methods, and the resulting outcomes" (p. 467).

After the occupational response has been made and its results manifest, the person needs to evaluate its quality. Because the occupational response is a consequence of the desire, demand, and press for mastery, the criterion used to assess the quality of the occupational response is *relative mastery*. This term emphasizes the fact that individuals experience mastery uniquely, relative to how well they feel their occupational response met the occupational challenge within the context of their occupational roles. OA proposes four criteria by which people evaluate their relative mastery: "efficiency (use of time, energy, resources); effectiveness (the extent to which the desired goal was achieved); satisfaction to self; and satisfaction to society" (Schultz 2009, p. 467). Each criterion is evaluated as negative, neutral, or positive. The same evaluation standards are used to make a judgment about the adaptiveness of the overall occupational response. Using adaptation terms, these three standards are labeled *disadaptive* (negative), *homeostasis* (neutral), and *adaptive* (positive). A response can be considered adaptive when the occupational challenge is overcome or met with mastery and competence. Responses are evaluated as disadaptive when they do not overcome the occupational challenge, often leaving the person feeling "stuck" and "unable to perform occupations and transact with the occupational environment with mastery and competence" (Grajo 2019, p. 637).

For an occupational response to become an adaptive response, it must lead to the ability to generalize. This process requires memory and reflection. Positive or negative evaluation of occupational responses can lead to integration of that response. Memories of occupational responses that led to positive results can be stored in memory as strategies that could potentially be useful in the future. Similarly, occupational responses that were evaluated negatively can prompt a person to reflect upon why they obtained the particular outcome and what might be done differently in the future in a similar situation. Schkade and Schultz (2003) clarified that "it is not skill mastery that produces generalization, but rather the adaptive capacity put to use... Without the adaptive capacity to anticipate outcomes, the individual is left with an array of specific skills whose applicability is specific rather than general" (p. 207). Adaptive capacity is a person's "ability to perceive the need to change, modify, or refine a variety of responses to occupational challenges" (Grajo 2019, p. 638). He likened adaptive capacity to having tools in a toolbox, questioning whether the person has sufficient tools to address occupational challenges that arise for them. As people generalize from specific instances, they add to their toolbox!

In summary, OA provides a conceptual framework for understanding how people respond and adapt to their environment. It conceptualizes people as occupational beings with a desire for mastery and environments as contexts that place demands for mastery. When in transaction, these produce a press for mastery that creates occupational roles, with their internal and external expectations, occupational challenges, and occupational responses underpinned by internal adaptive responses. In response to occupational challenges, they prepare with adaptive energy and respond from their unique adaptive gestalt. In the section that follows, we provide a brief overview of the principles that provide a foundation for using OA as an intervention process.

HISTORICAL DESCRIPTION OF THE MODEL'S DEVELOPMENT

The Occupational Adaptation Model (OAM) was developed by the occupational therapy faculty at Texas Woman's University in the United States as a framework upon which to build their research program and their Doctor of Philosophy in Occupational Therapy program. As Schultz (2009) explained, "One of the group's challenges was to name and frame how the program would contribute to the discipline and practice of occupational therapy". According to Schkade and Schultz (2003), the faculty decided that the focus of their research program should be the concepts of occupation and adaptation, as these two concepts were "historically important and central to occupational therapy" (p. 183). Consequently, their theoretical frame of reference was labeled *Occupational Adaptation*. In the years from 1994 (when the doctoral program was established) to 2007, 30 students graduated from the program (Schultz 2009).

It appears that the faculty at the university approached their research under the umbrella of occupational adaptation in different ways, with some faculty using a qualitative grounded theory methodology (Schkade and Schultz gave the examples of Spencer et al. 1998; Spencer and Davidson 1998; Spencer et al. 1999; White 1998). In their research, Schkade and Schultz became known for their theoretical work on occupational adaptation, which they continued because they were "asked to develop the group's conceptualization of occupational adaptation into the perspective that would be the core of the doctoral program" (Schultz 2009, p. 463). Anne Henderson, Lela Llorens, and Kathlyn Reed were asked to provide ongoing consultation into this process. According to Schultz (2009), OA was introduced as a frame of reference in 1992 and then, in 2003, as an "overarching theory for occupational therapy practice and research" (p. 463).

Emphasizing the significance of the historical inheritance of these ideas upon which OA is based, Schultz (2009) stated that "the intellectual heritage of this theory dates back to the writings of William Dunton (1913) and Adolf Meyer (1922)" (p. 463). The other, more recent, occupational therapy writer whose work reportedly influenced OA was Mary Reilly. Her concept of the importance of mastery to the health and well-being of humans is a central concept in OA.

Also emphasizing the occupational therapy heritage of OA, Schkade and Schultz (1992) listed four theories they claimed had "similarity with the proposed construct of occupational adaptation" (p. 830). These were Gilfoyle, Grady, and Moore's spatiotemporal adaptation (1990), a model of adaptation through occupation by Reed (1984), Kielhofner's Model of Human Occupation (1985), and a model of occupation by Nelson (1988). However, they did not outline what aspects of these models had similarities with OA, and how.

At the time of the first edition of this book, and compared with some other models reviewed in this book, OA had not changed very much since its early presentations in 1992. However, more recently Grajo (2017; 2019) has reconceptualized Schkade and Schultz's occupational adaptation process. While remaining true to the original theory, this reconceptualization uses much more contemporary language and emphasizes two aspects of occupational adaptation: as a normative, internal process and as an intervention process.

SUMMARY

OA emphasizes that it focuses on occupational adaptation rather than occupational performance. It distinguishes between occupational performance as an observable, behavioral outcome that may or may not result in occupational adaptation, which is an internal process. OA assumes people's desire for mastery transacts with the environment's demand for mastery, creating a press for mastery. This press, in turn, creates an occupational challenge. People can respond to this challenge adaptively by generating a response, evaluating that response, and then integrating the response into their repertoire of potential responses to use and adapt in the future. Integrating the response allows the person to generalize from a specific instance. Because people usually deal with multiple occupational challenges simultaneously, the process of occupational adaptation operates rapidly and repeatedly.

MEMORY AID

See Box 3.3.

BOX 3.3 ■ OAM Memory Aid

What roles does this person have?
What occupational challenges is this person currently facing in these roles?

For Each Occupational Challenge:

- How is this person's desire for mastery contributing to these?
- How is the environment's demand for mastery contributing to these?
- How are the desire and demand for mastery combining to generate a press for mastery that is creating these occupational challenges?

What occupational role expectations will be affected by these occupational challenges, and how will they be affected?

For Each Role:

- Could these current role expectations be changed so that they can be fulfilled successfully? If so, how (changes to person and/or environment)?

Occupational responses

- What occupational responses are required to enable the person to fulfill their role expectations in the relevant environment?
- How well is the person generating, evaluating, and integrating these occupational responses? If needed, what could be done to improve this process?

MAJOR WORKS

Grajo LC. Occupational adaptation. In: Hinojoa J, Kramer P. *Perspectives on Human Occupation: Theories Underlying Practice.* 2nd ed. F.A. Davis Company; 2017:287–311.

Grajo LC. Theory of Occupational Adaptation. In: Boyt Schell BA, Gillen G, Scaffa M, eds. *Willard & Spackman's Occupational Therapy.* 13th ed. Lippincott Williams & Wilkins; 2019:633–642.

Schkade JK, McClung M. *Occupational Adaptation in Practice: Concepts and Cases.* Slack; 2001.

Schkade JK, Schultz S. Occupational adaptation: toward a holistic approach to contemporary practice, part 1. *Am J Occup Ther.* 1992 Sep;46(9):829–837. doi:10.5014/ajot.46.9.829

Schkade JK, Schultz S. Occupational adaptation. In: Kramer P, Hinosa J, Royeen C, eds. *Perspectives in Human Occupation.* Lippincott Williams & Wilkins; 2003:181–221.

Schultz S. Theory of Occupational Adaptation. In: Crepeau EB, Cohn ES, Boyt Schell BA, eds. *Willard & Spackman's Occupational Therapy.* 11th ed. Lippincott Williams & Wilkins; 2009:462–475.

Schultz S, Schkade JK. Occupational adaptation: toward a holistic approach to contemporary practice, part 2. *Am J Occup Ther.* 1992 Oct;46(10):917–926. doi:10.5014/ajot.46.10.917

Schultz S, Schkade JK. Adaptation. In: Christiansen C, Baum C, eds. *Occupational Therapy: Enabling Function and Well-Being,* 2nd ed. Slack; 1997:458–481.

Conclusion

In this chapter we reviewed three occupational therapy models of practice: the AOTA's Operational Performance Model (OPM), the Operational Performance Model (Australia) (OPM(A), and the Theory of Occupational Adaptation (OA), also known as the Occupational Adaptation Model (OAM). The OPM and OPM(A) come from the tradition of occupational therapy theory that detailed the internal capacities affecting people's occupational performance. Both models are structured to include (1) occupational performance areas relating to self-care and maintenance, work and productivity, and play and leisure (to which the OPM(A) adds rest), and (2) occupational performance components/capacities, and they both emphasize the importance of occupational roles. Contrasting these two models helps highlight the conceptual shifts that have occurred in occupational therapy at different times in its history. The OPM(A) can also be seen to forecast the current focus on a holistic, transactional understanding of occupation.

The OAM centers on occupational adaptation as opposed to occupational performance. The concepts of occupation and adaptation are central to the OAM. OA assumes that people, as occupational beings, desire mastery of the environment and that the environment demands it. Their interaction produces a press for mastery that creates occupational roles and their internal and external expectations. These generate occupational challenges and occupational responses. Adaptation occurs when this process is internalized and generalized.

References

Chapparo C, Ranka J. The Occupational Performance Model (Australia): a description of constructs and structure. In: Chapparo C, Ranka J, eds. *Occupational Performance Model (Australia): Monograph 1*. Occupational Performance Network; 1997:1–23.

Chapparo C, Ranka J, Nott M. Occupational Performance Model (Australia): a description of constructs, structure and propositions. In: Curtin M, Egan M, Adams J, eds. *Occupational Therapy for People Experiencing Illness, Injury or Impairment: Promoting Occupation and Participation*. 7th ed. Elsevier; 2017:134–147.

Department of National Health and Welfare (DNHW) and Canadian Association of Occupational Therapists (CAOT). *Guidelines for the Client-Centred Practice of Occupational Therapists*. Cat. H39-33/1983E; 1983.

Dunton W. Occupation as a therapeutic measure. *Med Rec*. 1913;3:388–389.

Friedland J. Occupational therapy and rehabilitation: an awkward alliance. *Am J Occup Ther*. 1998 May;52(5):373–380. doi:10.5014/ajot.52.5.373

Gilfoyle E, Grady A, Moore J. *Children Adapt*. Slack; 1990.

Grajo LC. Occupational adaptation. In: Hinojoa J, Kramer P. *Perspectives on Human Occupation: Theories Underlying Practice*. 2nd ed. F.A. Davis Company; 2017:287–311.

Grajo LC. Theory of Occupational Adaptation. In: Boyt Schell BA, Gillen G, Scaffa M, eds. *Willard & Spackman's Occupational Therapy*. 13th ed. Lippincott Williams & Wilkins; 2019:633–642.

Hinojoa J, Kramer P. *Perspectives on Human Occupation: Theories Underlying Practice*. 2nd ed. F.A. Davis Company; 2017.

Hooper B, Wood W. Pragmatism and structuralism in occupational therapy: the long conversation. *Am J Occup Ther*. 2002 Jan-Feb;56(1):40–50. doi:10.5014/ajot.56.1.40

Kielhofner G. *A Model of Human Occupation: Theory and Application*. Lippincott Williams & Wilkins; 1985.

Lehman BJ, David DM, Gruber JA. Rethinking the biopsychosocial model of health: understanding health as a dynamic system. *Social & Personality Psychology Compass*. 2017 Aug;11(8):e12328. doi:10.1111/spc3.12328

Meyer A. The philosophy of occupational therapy. *Arch Occup Ther*. 1922;1:1–10.

Nelson DL. Occupation: form and performance. *Am J Occup Ther*. 1988 Oct;42(10):633–641. doi:10.5014/ajot.42.10.633

Pedretti LW. Occupational performance: a model for practice in physical dysfunction. In: Pedretti LW, ed. *Occupational Therapy: Practice Skills for Physical Dysfunction*. 4th ed. Mosby; 1996:3–12.

Pedretti LW, Early MB. Occupational performance and models of practice for physical dysfunction. In: Pedretti LW, Early MB, eds. *Occupational Therapy: Practice Skills for Physical Dysfunction*. 5th ed. Mosby; 2001:3–12.

Reed K. *Models of Practice in Occupational Therapy*. Lippincott Williams & Wilkins; 1984.

Reed K. An annotated history of the concepts used in occupational therapy. In: Christiansen CH, Baum MC, Bass-Haugen J, eds. *Occupational Therapy: Performance, Participation and Well-being*. 3rd ed. Slack; 2005:567–626.

Reilly M. Occupational therapy can be one of the greatest ideas of 20th century medicine (1961 Slagle Lecture). *Am J Occup Ther*. 1962 Jan-Feb;16:1–9.

Schkade JK, McClung M. *Occupational Adaptation in Practice: Concepts and Cases*. Slack; 2001.

Schkade JK, Schultz S. Occupational adaptation: toward a holistic approach to contemporary practice, part 1. *Am J Occup Ther*. 1992 Sep;46(9):829–837. doi:10.5014/ajot.46.9.829

Schkade JK, Schultz S. Occupational adaptation. In: Kramer P, Hinosa J, Royeen C, eds. *Perspectives in Human Occupation*. Lippincott Williams & Wilkins, 2003:181–221.

Schultz S. Theory of Occupational Adaptation. In: Crepeau EB, Cohn ES, Boyt Schell BA, eds. *Willard & Spackman's Occupational Therapy*. 11th ed. Lippincott Williams & Wilkins; 2009:462–475.

Schultz S, Schkade JK. Occupational adaptation: toward a holistic approach to contemporary practice, part 2. *Am J Occup Ther*. 1992 Oct;46(10):917–926. doi:10.5014/ajot.46.10.917

Spencer J, Davidson H. The Community Adaptive Planning Assessment: a clinical tool for documenting future planning with clients. *Am J Occup Ther*. 1998 Jan;52(1):19–30. doi:10.5014/ajot.52.1.19

Spencer J, Daybell PJ, Eschenfelder V, Khalaf R, Pike JM, Woods-Pettitti M. Contrasts in perspectives on work: an exploratory qualitative study based on the concept of adaptation. *Am J Occup Ther*. 1998 Jun;52(6):474–484. doi:10.5014/ajot.52.6.474

Spencer J, Hersch G, Eschenfelder V, Fournet J, Murray-Gerzik M. Outcomes of protocol-based and adaptation-based occupational therapy interventions for low-income elderly persons on a transitional unit. *Am J Occup Ther*. 1999 Mar-Apr;53(2):159–170. doi:10.5014/ajot.53.2.159

White VK. Ethnic differences in the wellness of elderly persons. *Occup Ther Health Care*. 1998;11(3):1–15. doi:10.1080/J003v11n03_01

CHAPTER 4

Ecological Models

CHAPTER CONTENTS

Person-Environment-Occupation Model   67
Main Concepts and Definitions of Terms   67
Historical Description of the Model's
   Development   71
Summary   72
Memory Aid   72
Major Works   73

Ecology of Human Performance Model   73
Main Concepts and Definitions of Terms   73
Interventions   75
Historical Description of the Model's
   Development   76
Summary   76
Memory Aid   77

Major Works   78

**Person-Environment-Occupation-
Performance Model   78**
Main Concepts and Definitions of Terms   78
The PEOP Occupational Therapy Process   80
Historical Description of the Model's
   Development   82
Summary   83
Memory Aid   83
Major Works   85

Conclusion   85

References   85

This chapter includes three models that center on the mutually influencing contributions of person, environment, and occupation to occupational performance. These models are the Person-Environment-Occupation (PEO) model by Law and others (1996); the Ecology of Human Performance (EHP) model (Dunn 2007; Dunn et al. 1994; Dunn et al. 2003); and the Person-Environment-Occupation-Performance (PEOP) model (Baum and Christiansen 2005, 2015; Christiansen and Baum 1991, 1997). The assumption underlying these models is that occupational performance is the product of the "goodness of fit" (Brown 2019) among person, environment, and occupation.

During the 1990s, a time of great proliferation of occupational therapy models, there was a concern that the contribution of the environment was not receiving adequate attention in occupational therapy, compared to the well-established focus on the person. At the time, occupational therapy was still emerging from its post-war mechanistic period, in which occupational performance problems were attributed to failures in the capacities of individuals and attention centered on remediating them. However, a feature of the intellectual climate of this time was awareness that people's lives are steeped in environmental conditions. The three models included in this chapter have been referred to by Brown (2019) as *ecological models*, which "draw heavily [on] social science theory that describe[s] person-environment interactions (Bronfenbrenner 1979; Gibson 1986; Lawton 1982; Csikszentmihalyi 1990)" (p. 623). Brown also explained that these models were influenced by the disability rights movements that emphasized the disabling effects of environments that form a barrier to occupational performance.

Person-Environment-Occupation Model

The first ecological model we present in this chapter is the Person-Environment-Occupation (PEO) model (Law et al. 1996). As the name suggests, the major concepts in this model of practice are person, environment, and occupation, which, when considered together, provide a way of understanding occupational performance. The concept of person-environment-occupation fit outlines the relationship among these different elements. When the three "fit" together well, it enhances occupational performance. However, when there is poor alignment among the three, occupational performance is reduced.

MAIN CONCEPTS AND DEFINITIONS OF TERMS

This model of practice was based on the literature on human ecology at the time of its publication. Human ecology is concerned with the relationship between human beings and their environment. As is evident in the models reviewed in this book, attention to the relationship between person and environment was a consistent feature in publications about occupational therapy models during the 1990s (both those developed during this time and the 1990s versions of those with multiple editions). This 1990s emphasis on understanding the person in the context of their environments probably represents the crystallizations of ideas that had been percolating during the 1970s and 1980s. It constitutes a move away from a biomedical model of health to a biopsychosocial model, where individuals are seen within their broader context (the broader systems that surround them).

PEO conceptualizes the relationship between the person and the environment as "transactive" (Law et al. 1996, p. 10) rather than interactive. The distinction between these two concepts relates to whether person and environment are conceptualized as distinct entities that could be studied separately or whether they should be examined together. An interactive approach would take the former position and consider the two as separate entities that are able to be measured separately and that influence the other in a cause-and-effect way. As Law et al. explained, "An interactive approach allows behaviour to be predicted and controlled, by influencing change at the level of an individual or environmental characteristic" (p. 10). In contrast, a transactive approach presents the person and environment as interdependent and proposes that a person's behavior cannot be separated from the context within which it occurs (including its temporal, physical, and psychological aspects). Therefore, from a transactive perspective, occupational performance is a context-, person-, and occupation-specific process. That is, it is the result of specific people doing particular things at certain times and places.

The relationship between person and environment is understood to be mutually influencing. As Law et al. (1996) stated, "a person's contexts are continually shifting and as contexts change, the behaviour necessary to accomplish a goal also changes" (p. 10). Therefore, rather than person and environment being examined separately, in a transactive approach an *event* becomes the unit of study. As such, the observable features of the environment in which the event took place would be investigated as well as the event's meaning to those participating in the event. This process provides for a rich understanding of the interconnectedness of person and environment and helps provide an understanding of how a person's behavior shapes and is shaped by the environment.

The distinction made within this model between interactive and transactive approaches to the person–environment relationship is important to understand because the two-dimensional diagram most associated with this model of three overlapping circles (person, environment, and occupation) could be misconstrued as representing an interactive rather than transactive approach. However, in its published form, a three-dimensional atom-like diagram was used (Fig. 4.1), which presents occupational performance as the nucleus of the transactional whole.

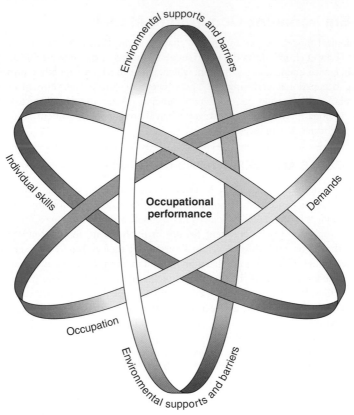

Fig. 4.1 Person-Environment-Occupation atom diagram. (From Law M, Cooper B, Strong S, Stewart D, Rigby P, Letts L. The Person-Environment-Occupation model: a transactive approach to occupational performance. *Can J Occup Ther.* 1996 Apr;63(1):9–23. doi:10.1177/000841749606300103. Reprinted with permission of CAOT Publications ACE.)

The diagram shows three interconnected components—environmental supports and barriers, individual skills, and occupational demands—surrounding occupational performance. Occupational performance is the "outcome of the transaction of the person, environment and occupation. It is defined as the dynamic experience of a person engaged in purposeful activities and tasks within an environment." (Law et al. 1996, p. 16). We encourage readers to keep the image of a transactional whole in the forefront of their minds as we discuss each dimension of the model.

The first element of the model that we explore is *person*. A biopsychosocial understanding of the person is evident in discussions in which Law et al. (1996) explain that occupational performance can be measured both objectively and subjectively. That is, there are features that can be observed and recorded in an objective way as well as features that relate to the experiences of the performer. The authors advocated that the latter be measured through methods such as self-report.

The changing nature of subjective experience and views of self is central to the concept of person in this model. The person is presented as "a dynamic, motivated and ever-developing being, constantly interacting with the environment" (p. 17). People change over time as the environments surrounding them change. They change in their attributes, characteristics, abilities, and skills and in how they think and feel about themselves. Their sense of who they are and what they are capable of develops and changes as they interact with the specific environments that surround them.

Consistent with this richly connected and contextualized view of the person is a broad definition of *environment*. As Law et al. (1996) stated, "the broad definition gives equal importance to the considerations of the environment" (p. 16). While occupational therapists have traditionally emphasized the influence of the physical environment on what people do and how they do it, this model makes explicit that a range of environmental considerations are equally important in influencing human behaviour and activity. While this broad concept of the environment is consistent with other models published in the 1990s, its uniqueness lies in its emphasis on the transactive relationship between the environment and the person. The only other model that emphasized this degree of interconnectedness at the time was the Ecology of Human Performance model (Dunn et al. 1994), which is the next model presented in this chapter.

The PEO model outlines five aspects of the context surrounding the person—cultural, socioeconomic, institutional, physical, and social—that shape and are shaped by that person. For example, culture shapes what people believe and how they see the world. This, in turn, shapes how they think about themselves and what they want to do and/or are expected to do. However, individuals' views of the world and of themselves are also dependent upon the degree to which they internalize the views of the culture and the people surrounding them. Their socioeconomic circumstances will also influence their perception of what they can and cannot do as well as their access to resources. Just as people grow and age and change in their skills, abilities, character, and experiences, so too are their contexts and circumstances likely to change over the course of their lives. Environments can change because people physically relocate; change their roles, habits, and routines; or change their social and cultural groupings, etc.; or because local, national, and world circumstances change. For example, the environment surrounding a person living at the beginning of the 20th century will differ greatly from that of a person living during the 21st century.

The third aspect of the model considers what people do within their environmental contexts. While this is called *occupation* in the model's name, Law et al. (1996) considered three aspects of human action—activity, task, and occupation—under this category. They presented these three concepts as "nested within each other" (p. 16) and claimed they drew upon the work of Christiansen and Baum (1991) in their categorization (note: Christiansen and Baum's recent hierarchy does not use the word *activity* at all, possibly because there is a lack of consensus about whether activity is a component of a task or vice versa). Commencing with the smallest of the three, *activity* was defined in the PEO as "a singular pursuit in which a person engages as part of his/her daily occupational experience" and considered "the basic unit of a task" (p. 16). They gave the example of the act of handwriting. Next, *task* was defined as "a set of purposeful activities in which a person engages" and could be represented by, for example, "the obligation to write a report" (p. 16). Finally, *occupation* was referred to as "groups of self-directed, functional tasks and activities in which a person engages over the lifespan" (p. 16). To continue with the same example, Law et al. suggested that occupation would be "a managerial position requiring an individual to engage in frequent report writing" (p. 16), which might constitute one of their professional activities.

Law et al. (1996) further defined *occupations* (plural) as "those clusters of activities and tasks in which the person engages in order to meet his/her intrinsic needs for self-maintenance, expression and fulfilment" (p. 16) and explained that they are linked to roles and conducted in multiple environments. This definition emphasizes that self-maintenance, expression, and fulfillment are considered intrinsic needs and that people engage in occupations within the context of their specific roles and environments. It is these roles and environments that shape the process and purpose of occupations for a particular person.

Occupational performance results from the interconnectedness of people, what they are aiming to do, and where it will be done. However, the rich connections among these three factors are evident when realizing that even when individuals make decisions about what to do, these decisions are shaped by the broader context in which they live. A complex process occurs in which people determine the purpose of occupations in their lives. This process is shaped by their perceptions, goals, responsibilities, and desires and the demands of the context in which they live. In a reciprocal way, how they think about themselves and what they do also influence their environments.

The concept of the person-environment-occupation fit is central to the model. The degree of congruence among the three elements determines occupational performance. Fig. 4.2 represents this process. The three circles overlap to different extents, resulting in differences in occupational performance that are represented by the section where all three elements overlap. As Law et al. (1996) stated, "the outcome of greater compatibility is therefore represented as more optimal occupational performance" (p. 17). When the congruence among them diminishes, occupational performance is impeded. The goal of occupational therapy is to improve any reduced occupational performance by facilitating or enhancing the fit among person, environment, and occupation.

As evident in the diagram, these overlapping circles come from a cross section of the diagram used to represent the temporal aspects of occupational performance throughout the lifespan. Fig. 4.2 shows a tube of ongoing development with its transactions at different times of life. The overlap of the three circles representing occupational performance differs at various times in a person's life. This figure indicates that occupational performance changes over time and throughout the lifespan, as the relationships among person, environment, and occupation change.

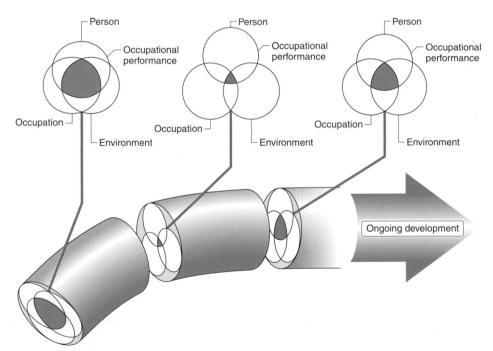

Fig. 4.2 Person-Environment-Occupation lifespan diagram. (From Law M, Cooper B, Strong S, Stewart D, Rigby P, Letts L. The Person-Environment-Occupation model: a transactive approach to occupational performance. *Can J Occup Ther*. 1996 Apr;63(1):9–23. doi:10.1177/000841749606300103. Reprinted with permission of CAOT Publications ACE.)

Written at a time when ideas from a systems approach and the biopsychosocial model of health were prominent, the PEO model emphasized that occupational performance was person, environment, and occupation specific and that the three could not be considered separately. Consequently, intervention could be targeted at any one or more of the three elements, as a change in one would be expected to lead to a change in the others. However, it is important to note that a transactive understanding of the relationship among the three components means that, while a change is expected, the exact nature of that change *cannot be predicted*.

At the time, Law et al. (1996) listed four advantages of using the PEO model:

1. It enables people to select from and use interventions that are directed at person, occupation, and environment in different ways.
2. It provides a framework for using multiple paths to effect change.
3. It draws particular attention to interventions that address different levels of the environment and the importance of selecting and implementing interventions "in context."
4. By taking an ecological approach to the environment, it provides for the "use of a wider repertoire of well validated instruments of measure developed by other disciplines" (p. 18).

HISTORICAL DESCRIPTION OF THE MODEL'S DEVELOPMENT

There is a certain level of symmetry in placing a transactional model, which assumes action takes place within a certain context, within its specific historical and geographical context. This model was published in 1996, a decade in which occupational therapy models were commonly emphasizing occupational therapy's assumption that people should be understood in a holistic way. That is, they should be understood as both "whole" people (rather than just bodies) and people who live in specific contexts (their "whole" situation). Placed within the broader context of models of health, this decade was a time when a biopsychosocial understanding of health was becoming more established, in contrast to the biomedical understanding characteristic of the preceding period.

Law et al. (1996) claimed that the importance of the relationship between person and environment had been well recognized during the profession's early history but was not emphasized from the 1940s to the 1960s (a time that Reed, 2005, described as the mechanistic period and being characterized by the "forgetting" of many formative concepts). Law et al. summed up this view of the situation by saying, "Occupational performance results from the dynamic relationship among people, their occupations and roles, and the environments in which they live, work and play. There have, however, been few models of practice in the occupational therapy literature which discuss the theoretical and clinical applications of person–environment interaction" (p. 9). Presumably, the authors saw the need for occupational therapy to make explicit its contextualized understanding of human occupation.

The main article presenting this model appeared in the *Canadian Journal of Occupational Therapy* in 1996. In providing their rationale for the model, Law et al. (1996) argued that occupational therapy's "views on the relationship between occupation and the environment have altered" (p. 10), in that perspectives had moved away from the cause-and-effect assumptions inherent within a biomedical model of health and moved toward a more "transactive" (p. 10) understanding of occupational performance. They also provided a literature review, highlighting key publications that demonstrated "the importance of the environment in influencing behaviour and the use of the environment as a treatment modality in occupational therapy" (p. 13). They noted that this concern had been increasingly discussed from the mid-1980s to the mid-1990s. Thus they placed the model within the existing trends in occupational therapy.

This placing of the model within existing trends might suggest the authors were aiming to describe the theory and practice of occupational therapy at the time, rather than intending to shape it into a new understanding. (This is different from some other models reviewed in this book, which do appear to have the aim of shaping occupational therapy theory and practice in particular ways.) If this assumption is correct, it might help to explain why this model is so well known and used, despite having only been published in one major article. That is, it may have provided occupational therapists with a language and concepts for describing what they believed about their theory and practice related to occupation. Certainly, the concepts of person, environment, and occupation being interdependent and mutually influencing have become central to occupational therapy discourse about human action in the intervening years.

Law et al. (1996) also explained that "the previous medical orientation of practice has linked occupational therapy more naturally with other health professionals and not necessarily fostered interaction with social scientists, human geographers, architects and interior designers, interested in planning therapeutic and enabling environments" (p. 14). This is an interesting statement to reflect upon more than two decades later, when similar sentiments have been expressed by those advocating for an occupational science approach and changes in the healthcare context to incorporate a broader view of health and the proliferation of occupational therapists working in areas other than health.

SUMMARY

The PEO model presents the three major components of occupational therapy's domain of concern—person, environment, and occupation—and conceptualizes their relationship as transactive. This means they should not be considered separately but are considered mutually influencing, in that a change in any one or more domains leads to a change in the others. While change is expected, the model suggests the exact nature of the change cannot be predicted or controlled. The degree to which these three elements *fit* together influences occupational performance. That is, if the congruence among person-environment-occupation is high, occupational performance will be enhanced. If the fit is poor, occupational performance is reduced. The aim of occupational therapy is to facilitate occupational performance by intervening in any one or more of these areas to enhance the congruence among person, environment, and occupation.

MEMORY AID

See Box 4.1.

BOX 4.1 ■ Person-Environment-Occupation Model Memory Aid

- What events are relevant to this client? (What does this person need/want to do in the context of their life?)
  - What occupation is required?
  - Who will do it?
  - What does it mean to that person?
  - In what environment and under what circumstances will it be done?
- How are/have the cultural, socioeconomic, institutional, physical, and social environments shaping/shaped that perception?
- How are they performing those activities, tasks, and occupations (objective measures)?
- How do they experience performing those activities, tasks, and occupations (subjective measures)?
- What degree of congruence exists between:
  - The person's abilities, perceptions, and experiences
  - The cultural, socioeconomic, institutional, physical, and social environment
  - The activities, tasks, and occupations that are being/need to be performed?
- What combination of interventions might assist in increasing the congruence among person, environment, and occupation?
- Where could those interventions be targeted (person, environment, occupation)?

MAJOR WORKS

Law M, Cooper B, Strong S. The Person-Environment-Occupation Model: a transactive approach to occupational performance. *Can J Occup Ther*. 1996;63(1):9–23. doi:10.1177/000841749606300

Ecology of Human Performance Model

The Ecology of Human Performance (EHP) model (Dunn et al. 1994) conceptualizes the environment as an inseparable aspect of occupation; that is, it is the context within which people act and which shapes and is shaped by that action. It was published in 1994, two years before the PEO model was published. When reading about the EHP in this chapter, it is important to remember that many comments expressed, such as the need to expand the concept of the environment beyond the physical environment, have become embedded in occupational therapy thinking in the intervening three decades. Reading about the model's advocacy for an ecological understanding of human occupation should emphasize for readers how influential these ideas have been in occupational therapy. Another important point to make is that EHP uses the term *task* rather than *occupation*. Because the model aimed to address an interdisciplinary audience, the term *task* was intentionally used due to its perceived stability of meaning for this broader audience.

MAIN CONCEPTS AND DEFINITIONS OF TERMS

The EHP portrays the environment as the primary context within which performance needs to be understood. It is a lens through which all human performance should be viewed. According to Dunn et al. (1994), the term *ecology* refers to the "interrelationships of organisms and their environments" (p. 595), and the model emphasizes the interrelatedness of person, context, task, and performance. In the original 1994 publication, the authors stated, "the primary theoretical postulate fundamental to the EHP framework is that ecology, or the interaction between person and the environment, affects human behaviour and performance, and that performance cannot be understood outside of context" (p. 598). Thus context is central to human performance. Fig. 4.3 provides a diagrammatic representation of the EHP. In this model there are three important constructs—person, task, and context (initially called environment)—which contribute to an understanding of the fourth construct: human performance (Dunn 2007).

A central feature of this model is the primary importance to human performance of *environment* or *context*. The model conceptualizes the environment as the broader context that is integral to and shapes both the person and their task performance. This understanding of the environment has two aspects that need to be considered in more depth: (1) the environment includes more than just the physical environment; and (2) the environment has the capacity to shape task performance.

First, while the earlier publications of the model use the term *environment* (or *context-environment*), the authors articulated very clearly that the term is conceptualized very broadly and should not be limited to the physical environment. They stated that the concept of the environment should be expanded to include "physical, temporal, social, and cultural elements" (Dunn et al. 1994, p. 596). By expanding the definition of environment in this way, Dunn et al. emphasized the contribution that occupational therapists can make to an understanding of the interdependent relationship between the person and the environment. They claimed that a broad definition of environment helps make explicit the complexity of the person–environment relationship to a level that is beyond the scope of the work done by environmental psychologists (who mainly focused on the physical environment). In particular, a broader concept of the

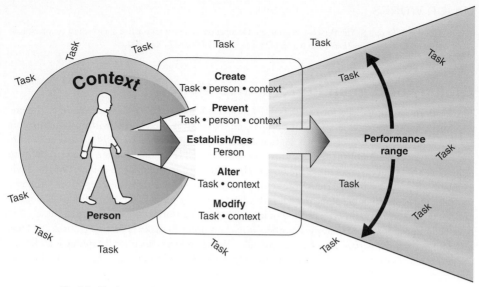

Fig. 4.3 Ecology of Human Performance based on Dunn, Brown & McQuigan, 1994.

environment allows occupational therapists to consider the meaning of the physical, temporal, social, and cultural environment to the person.

Second, while the influence of the environment on human performance has long been acknowledged in occupational therapy, the EHP model emphasizes that the environment also shapes both the person and the tasks in which that person engages. In a review of the social science literature on the effect of the environment, Dunn et al. (1994, p. 596) cited a range of different authors and the main emphasis of their work. These included:

- Bruner (1989), who conceptualized the environment as providing a context for the construction of the self
- Lawton (1982), who applied Murray's (1938) concept of environmental press, emphasizing that the demands of the environment influence a person's perceptions of their own competence
- Gibson's (1986) phenomenological approach to perception, whereby people's perceptions of objects in the environment are influenced by the opportunities the environment affords them

These are just a few of the ideas that influenced the EHP's concept of the importance of the environment in shaping how people view themselves and what they do.

As the focus of the model is the relationship between person and environment, the second construct we will discuss here is *person*. Dunn et al. (2003) stated that "the Ecology of Human Performance is an individually focused, client-centered framework. Individuals are seen as unique and complex" (p. 225). Personal variables contribute to the uniqueness of individuals. These are listed in the model as values, interests, and experiences, as well as sensorimotor, cognitive, and psychosocial skills. These personal variables influence both the selection of tasks and the quality of task performance. These personal variables are also continually influenced by people's continually changing contexts.

The third construct is *task*. The model takes the view that a multitude of tasks are potentially available to all people. However, an individual's *actual* repertoire of tasks is shaped by personal and environmental variables. Personal variables such as interests, values, perceptions, and experience as well as sensorimotor, cognitive, and psychosocial skills and abilities influence the selection of tasks in which the person participates. Environmental variables also influence task selection and performance. For example, some tasks might not be easily accessed in certain environments such as snow skiing in a temperate climate, while others might not be socially or culturally valued. In addition, people might engage in a certain selection of tasks because the context "requires" these tasks of them. Examples include tasks that are required to fulfill particular social roles. The specific sets of tasks in which people engage will depend on the unique relationship between them and their specific context. The EHP model refers to this set of tasks as the *performance range*, and people select from the tasks available to them in this range. The performance range is influenced by people's skills and abilities and the supports and barriers created by their context. As people and contexts change, so too do their performance ranges.

The final construct in the model is *human performance*. This is the result of the interaction among person, context, and task. All the factors discussed for each of these combine to result in human performance.

INTERVENTIONS

In addition to the four core constructs already discussed, the EHP model addresses five categories of interventions: establish/restore, alter, adapt, prevent, and create. These five alternatives for intervention relate variously to person, context, and task.

First, therapeutic interventions can aim to *establish* or *restore* an individual's skills and abilities. This intervention approach refers to either establishing skills that people have not previously developed or restoring skills and abilities they have lost, usually through acquiring a medical condition, injury, or disability. Dunn et al. (1994) made the point that restorative interventions are very common among occupational therapists working within a biomedical model, with its corrective emphasis. While these interventions target the individual's skills and abilities, Dunn et al. stressed that context can be important in these types of interventions and gave the example of how important predictable environments are in providing feedback for correcting motor behaviors.

The second way occupational therapists could intervene is to *alter* or *change* the environment. This intervention aims to create the best match between people and their environments and focuses on selecting a different environment rather than adapting the current environment (this is not to be confused with altering or making changes to the current environment). For example, they might select different environments that enable people to perform those tasks.

The third intervention alternative is to *adapt* the contextual features and/or task demands. Regarding contextual features, these could be enhanced or minimized to better match the person's abilities. Similarly, aspects of the task such as the sequence of steps, the tools used, the position required of the person, and the skills required of the person can be adapted to enable the person to participate in the task.

The fourth intervention alternative is to *prevent*. In this option, occupational therapists might aim to "prevent the occurrence or evolution of maladaptive performance in context" (Dunn et al. 1994, p. 604). This intervention strategy aims to prevent difficulties from arising. To do this, occupational therapists might address person, context, and/or task.

The final intervention option is called *create* and was described by Dunn et al. as "creating circumstances that promote more adaptable or complex performance in context" (p. 604). The authors stressed that this intervention does not assume the presence of a disability or that there is a problem that will interfere with performance.

HISTORICAL DESCRIPTION OF THE MODEL'S DEVELOPMENT

Like the PEO model, the EHP model was developed at a time when the profession was making more explicit its fundamental assumptions about the importance of the environment in occupational performance. In many ways, the 1990s could be seen as a time in occupational therapy's history in which the reductionism of the mechanistic period was increasingly being critiqued and many of occupational therapy's fundamental beliefs were being reaffirmed.

The EHP model was developed by the Department of Occupational Therapy at the University of Kansas, originally for three reasons outlined by Dunn (2007):

1. To produce a framework that would support and guide the scholarly work produced by that department
2. To provide a means for organizing their curriculum and communicating their perspectives to their students
3. Most importantly, according to Dunn, to develop a framework to support the planning of work conducted in conjunction with their interdisciplinary colleagues

According to Dunn, the EHP model was successful in supporting all three original aims. At the time the model was developed, the authors (Dunn et al. 1994) explained that, while the environment had been "a recurring theme in the occupational therapy literature" (p. 595), insufficient attention had been made to the influence of contextual features on human performance. Dunn (2007) also emphasized that, at the time, the context had also been neglected by other services as well as occupational therapy.

In the major publications on this model between 1994 and 2019, the model has undergone very little change. The major difference is really one of categorization, in that the original version of the model included "therapeutic intervention" as a fifth construct in the practice of occupational therapy (in addition to person, task, context, and occupational performance). While intervention was not listed as a separate construct in later versions of the model, the five different intervention strategies outlined in the earlier version—establish/restore, alter, adapt, prevent, and create—have remained an integral part of the model.

In discussing the development of the EHP model, Dunn (2007) emphasized the conscious decision not to use the term *occupation* in the model. This was because one of its original purposes was to provide a framework from which to work with colleagues outside the discipline of occupational therapy, and the authors thought the particular way occupational therapists use the term *occupation* could make this process difficult. Instead, the term *task* was used, as the developers were of the opinion that it had utility and a common understanding within everyday language. However, in the later publications, the concept of occupation, which had very much taken root in occupational therapy discourse by then, was discussed more overtly. For example, in explaining the choice to use the word *task* in a 2007 publication, Dunn emphasized that the "construct of occupation" (p. 128), whereby a person derives meaning from performance of a task in context, is important to understanding human performance.

While EHP has undergone little change or development over time, it has had a broad influence on occupational therapy. In 2007, Dunn stated that "One of the most helpful benefits of including context is that intervention options expand" (p. 128). Interestingly, the five intervention approaches Dunn et al. identified in 1994—establish/restore, adapt/modify, alter, prevent, and create—appear to have influenced the American Occupational Therapy Association's Occupational Therapy Practice Framework (AOTA 2002, 2008, 2014, 2020), as these five appear in that document as treatment planning and implementation strategies.

SUMMARY

The EHP model is an ecological model of occupational therapy that emphasizes the context through which task performance should be viewed. Whereas other models of practice in occupational therapy generally start with the person and focus on occupational performance in context, this model starts with context.

The model was first published in 1994 and has changed very little in the three major publications in which it has been presented. The primary focus of the model is the person in context. People in their contexts have a range of tasks available to them, and this range is influenced by both person and context. The role of occupational therapy is to identify this performance range of available tasks and determine whether it meets the needs of the person in that context.

MEMORY AID

See Box 4.2.

BOX 4.2 ■ Ecology of Human Performance Model Memory Aid

In this Situation:

- Who is the relevant person?
  - What are their experiences; interests; and sensorimotor, cognitive, and psychosocial skills (and how have these changed or how are they likely to change)?
  - In what ways does the context shape them or do they shape the context?
  - How do their abilities/skills/interests affect task selection and performance?
- What are the relevant contexts?
  - Temporal environment (e.g., age, life cycle, time in history)?
  - Physical environment?
  - Social environment?
  - Cultural environment?
  - How well do these match the person's abilities/interests/skills and the tasks that need to be done?
  - How are these contexts likely to change?
- What are the relevant tasks (sets of behaviors, could be components of occupation)?
  - What tasks are available to the person?
  - How well do the tasks match the person's abilities/skills/interests?
  - What tasks are available in the relevant contexts?

Intervention Planning:

Which intervention methods could be used to facilitate successful participation and where will they be aimed?

- Establish/restore
- Alter (different environment)
- Adapt/modify

- Prevent (anticipate problem)

- Create

Personal skills and abilities
Context (environmental variables)
Context (environmental variables)
Task (demands of)
Context (environmental variables)
Personal variables
Task Variables
Context (environmental variables)
Personal variables

- _____
- _____
- _____
- _____

MAJOR WORKS

Dunn W. Ecology of Human Performance model. In: Dunbar SB, ed. *Occupational Therapy Models for Intervention with Children and Families*. Slack; 2007:127–155.

Dunn W, Brown C, McGuigan A. The ecology of human performance: a framework for considering the effect of context. *Am J Occup Ther*. 1994 Jul;48(7):595–607. doi:10.5014/ajot.48.7.595

Dunn W, Brown C, Youngstrom MJ. Ecological model of occupation. In: Kramer P, Hinojosa J, Royeen CB, eds. *Perspectives in Human Occupation: Participation in Life*. Lippincott Williams & Wilkins; 2003:222–263.

Person-Environment-Occupation-Performance Model

The Person-Environment-Occupation-Performance (PEOP) ecological model (Baum et al. 2015) has changed markedly from edition to edition, with four editions in 1991, 1997, 2005, and 2015. In this chapter we present the fourth edition of the model (Baum et al. 2015; Baum et al. 2020). It was published in 2015 in the textbook *Occupational Therapy: Performance, Participation, and Well-Being* (Christansen et al. 2015), with an overview provided in Baum et al. (2015) and details of the components provided in the various chapters of the book. According to Baum et al. (2020), it draws upon "knowledge and evidence generated from occupational therapy science, neuroscience, environmental science and other biological and social sciences" (p. 88). Developments in these areas have enabled the PEOP model to develop its theoretical and scientific basis over time.

The PEOP model is described as a transactive systems model in which personal and environmental factors are conceived as influencing the performance of everyday occupations. (Readers will note that the word *transactive* was also used in the PEO model.) As with the other two models reviewed in this chapter, PEOP is an ecological model. As Baum et al. (2020) explained, making reference to the third edition, "it identifies three relevant domains of knowledge for occupational therapy practice, all of which interact to support the occupational performance of individuals, groups or populations: (1) the person, group or population factors (previously identified as intrinsic factors); (2) the environmental factors that include the situation and context, and relevant cultural, physical, social, policy and technological environments (previously identified as the extrinsic factors); and (3) the occupations of importance to the client's well-being (activities, tasks and roles)" (p. 87).

MAIN CONCEPTS AND DEFINITIONS OF TERMS

The fourth edition of the PEOP model is based on four concepts. The first is *collaboration*. The occupational therapy approach is essentially a cooperative one in which occupational therapists collaborate with clients to form goals that are meaningful and useful. A foundational assumption is that only the clients fully understand their situation, and occupational therapists should work with and be guided by them. The model acknowledges that collaboration might occur directly with people such as children, adults, and families, or in conjunction with others such as other health professionals, architects, employers, organizations, and entire communities. All of these can be considered *clients* if they are seeking the knowledge and skills of occupational therapists.

The second concept the model focuses on is *occupational performance*. The fourth edition defines occupational performance as "the doing of meaningful activities, tasks, and roles through complex interactions between the person and environment" (Baum et al. 2015, p. 52). Occupational performance occurs in connection with the people's occupational roles and their sociocultural environments and therefore has meaning and purpose as well as implications for self-identity.

The third concept is *systems perspective*. In dynamic systems theory, systems are able to self-organize, changing their components and the relationships among the components as required to maintain equilibrium. The components of the model—that is, the person environment and the occupational elements—are mutually influencing and connected in a dynamic whole. For example, when people engage in occupation, the process changes both the environment and the people in terms of their self-identity, their physical and cognitive capacities, and so forth. Similarly, characteristics of the environment will shape how people engage in and perform occupations.

The fourth concept guiding the PEOP model is *client centeredness*. Baum et al. (2020) stated that "the PEOP model provides a bridge from the biomedical model to a sociocultural model of health" (p. 88) in that, while recognizing the effect of impairments on performance and participation (biomedical), it also attends to the person in context. Occupational therapists must understand where people live, how they live their lives, and what they want and need to do. They often come to understand this by listening to people's stories about their lives. Through these narratives, they can collaboratively formulate goals that aim to enable people to live their lives as they need and want to.

As an ecological model, the PEOP model is concerned with the degree to which the person–environment fit supports or inhibits occupational participation, performance, and well-being. The ultimate goal is to facilitate an optimal person–environment fit. While person and environment are both discussed in detail as components of the model, this is done to contextualize the increased participation, occupational performance, and well-being that result from the valued outcomes of individuals, organizations, and populations.

The PEOP model consists of four components. As with all ecological models, it has person, environment, and occupation components; to these it adds a component known as the narrative. Fig. 4.4 shows the concepts of person and environment as two ellipses overlapping each other, influencing occupation, which is conceptualized in terms of participation, performance, and well-being.

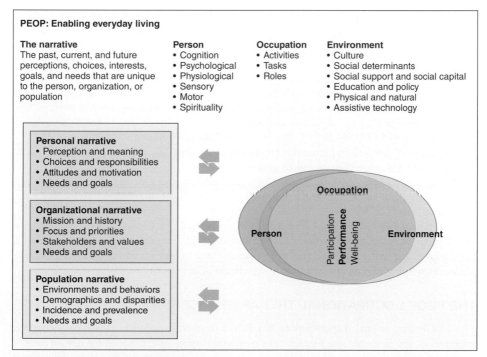

Fig. 4.4 Person-Environment-Occupation-Performance model. Christiansen CH, Baum CM, Bass-Haugen J. *Occupational Therapy: Performance, Participation and Well-Being.* 4th ed. Thorofare, NJ: Slack; 2015. Reprinted with permission from Slack.

The *narrative* is presented in the diagram as personal narratives, organizational narratives, and population narratives. These narratives provide a way of synthesizing information about clients' perspectives, values, and concerns. Essentially, it is the person's story that can tie together all the pieces of information an occupational therapist has gathered in a range of ways from a diversity of sources. Understanding the narrative is essential for collaboratively setting goals for occupational therapy. The PEOP model provides a framework for organizing information and a systematic approach to planning intervention for clients of all ages and life stages with a variety of occupational performance challenges. Using the PEOP model, occupational therapists are guided to plan interventions that center on people's life situations and enable them to perform the occupations that are necessary for living satisfying and meaningful lives in those contexts. The PEOP model uses a "top-down" approach in which the narrative of the person, organization, or population is generated first and is followed by valuation of aspects of the person and environment that enable or impede occupational performance. The narrative provides the guiding force for what is done and how it is done.

The person factors that contribute to or limit occupational performance are explored in detail in the PEOP model. Baum et al. (2020) detailed these as:

- "physiological characteristics such as strength, endurance, flexibility, activity levels, stress, sleep nutrition and health;
- cognitive dimensions including organization, reasoning, attention, awareness, executive function and memory — all necessary for task performance;
- sensory/perceptual characteristics including somatosensory, olfactory, gustatory, visual, auditory, proprioceptive and tactile;
- motor functions, including motor control, motor planning (praxis), motor learning and postural control;
- psychological factors including emotional state (affect), self-concept, self-esteem, sense of identity, self-efficacy and theory of mind (social awareness); and
- spiritual dimensions, which include beliefs and practices that influence personal meaning" (p. 89).

The environmental factors include:

- Social determinants of health, including social support, which could be emotional, practical, instrumental, or informational, and social capital in terms of interpersonal relationships, social receptivity, laws, education, and policies
- The cultural environment, including "values, beliefs, customs and use of time"
- Features of physical and natural environments, including "physical properties, tools, [and] geography, to reign climate and air quality"
- Assistive technology, which includes "personal technology and design". The rapid development in digital technology can also be harnessed to facilitate occupational performance and participation (p. 90)

In summary, the PEOP model is an ecological, transactive systems model concerned with the contribution of occupational, personal, and environmental factors to occupational performance, participation, and well-being. Occupational therapists come to understand this through the clients' narratives, whereby clients can be persons, organizations, or populations.

THE PEOP OCCUPATIONAL THERAPY PROCESS

The PEOP occupational therapy process has four components: narrative, assessment/evaluation, intervention, and outcomes (see Fig. 4.5). The *narrative* phase commences with the development of an occupational profile and occupational history. The purpose of these is to elicit a story of the client's

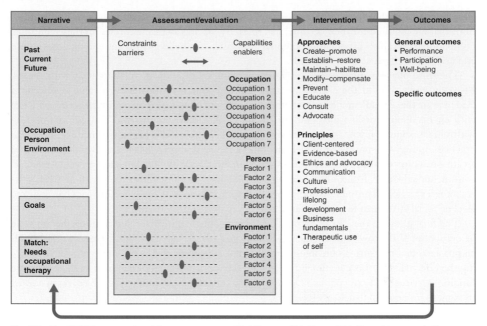

Fig. 4.5 The PEOP occupational therapy process. Christiansen CH, Baum CM, Bass-Haugen J. *Occupational Therapy: Performance, Participation and Well-Being.* 4th ed. Slack; 2015. Reprinted with permission from Slack.

life context, thereby providing a rich tapestry within which to interpret the meaning and importance of information as it is gained. Through the occupational profile and history, occupational therapists learn about the circumstances of people, organizations, and populations; their current interest and projects; their past experiences and occurrences; and the futures they are working toward. For individuals, this can include the interests, social activities, and responsibilities for work, self, and home management tasks, as well as their understanding of any medical and health challenges they are facing and options for interventions. Once an occupational profile and history has been developed, client goals are collaboratively determined that are appropriate and achievable in the context of their lives. Baum et al. (2020) proposed using a temporal progression for goals, commencing with longer-term goals. By establishing these goals first, the steps required to achieve them can be identified as short-term goals. Goals must be considered in terms of the narrative understanding developed. As Baum et al. stated, "by knowing the person's interests, skills, values, roles, traditions, habits and routines, it is possible to help identify goals that are meaningful" (p. 90). When considering potential goals, occupational therapists should be aware of the propensity for cultural stereotypes to shape assumptions and of the experiences of marginalized groups.

The final aspect of the narrative phase of the process is to review the degree to which client goals can be addressed by occupational therapy. Baum et al. (2020) referred to this as "the match between the client's goals and the occupational therapy approach" (p. 90). When there is poor alignment, appropriate referrals to other professionals and resources can be made. When they match well, occupational therapists move to the next phase: assessment/evaluation.

In the *assessment/evaluation* phase, results relating to occupation, person, and environment are each placed on a continuum from constraints/barriers to capabilities/enablers. Assessments are chosen to explore the effects of these on people's performance of the activities, tasks, and occupations that are required for their occupational roles. By placing assessment roles on these continua, occupational therapists can identify potential problems and challenges on one end of a continuum and areas of strength at the other end.

The third phase is *intervention*. Intervention plans are developed collaboratively with clients, based on knowledge of the client's narrative and assessment results. A high value is placed on evidence in the PEOP model. Occupational therapists have a responsibility to share evidence with clients about possible interventions. Baum et al. (2020) emphasized that communicating with clients about evidence for intervention plans represents the highest principles of ethical practice. As Fig. 4.5 shows, the model advocates a range of approaches to intervention including create-promote, establish-restore, maintain-habilitate, modify-compensate, prevent, educate, consult, and advocate. Many of these approaches are used to guide direct intervention, while others represent a health promotion and prevention approach as well as advocating for change as the level of social structures to remove barriers to occupational performance.

The final phase of the PEOP occupational therapy process involves determining the outcome of occupational therapy and whether the client goals have been achieved. Baum et al. (2020) emphasized that measuring outcomes is important for showing clients their progress and displaying the effectiveness of occupational therapy interventions to stakeholders such as those who are funding services and the public. Demonstrating effectiveness publicly enables occupational therapy to influence policies.

HISTORICAL DESCRIPTION OF THE MODEL'S DEVELOPMENT

The PEOP model is presented within the context of a larger text, *Occupational Therapy: Performance, Participation and Well-Being* (Christiansen et al. 2015). This textbook relates to occupational therapy more generally and takes the reader through the fundamental assumptions of the profession relating to occupation before presenting the model. Thus the PEOP model forms one part of Christiansen and Baum's broader conceptualization of occupation and occupational therapy.

The model commenced its development in 1985 (Baum and Christiansen 2005) and has been published in 1991, 1997, 2005, and 2015. The impetus for developing the model was the largely biomedical framing of knowledge that limited occupational therapists practicing in a holistic way that focused on enabling people to improve the quality of their lives. As Baum et al. (2015) explained, "at that time, the most influential text books in the field were continuing to organize their content using a biomedical approach that resembled the diagnosis and pathology-focused approach of allopathic medicine" (p. 50). In contrast, the PEOP model provided a framework based on health and well-being.

The distinction between occupation, performance, and occupational performance is evident in all four editions of the model, with the fourth edition presenting occupation as contributing to participation and well-being, as well as performance. The distinction between these concepts can be traced back to the model's use of Nelson's 1988 work, in which he distinguished between occupational form and performance. Christiansen (1991) stated, "all the elements comprising the context of the occupation are what Nelson (1988) terms *the form* of occupation. Occupational performance consists of *the doing* of occupation." (p. 27, italics in original.) In an adaptation of Nelson's work, Christiansen conceptualized occupational form as "the objective context of occupation consisting of: materials, environmental surround, other humans involved, temporal dimension, and sociocultural reality derived from social or cultural consensus" (p. 26).

In the first edition of the model, a binary distinction appears to have been made between performance and Christiansen's concept of adaptation of occupational form, the latter relating to what is done, the context in which it is done, and the meaning of the doing to an individual. In this way, the first edition appears to have distinguished between performance and a broad conceptualization of occupational form, with the latter being ascribed meaning by an individual and occurring within a particular content.

In the second edition, a trio of concepts was presented. These were person, environment, and occupational performance. This version emphasized that the performance of occupation is affected by a complex array of factors that influence performance, "as well as the many dimensions of occupation" (Christiansen and Baum 1997b, p. 49). These dimensions of occupation were discussed in terms of occupational performance and form, with Christiansen and Baum stating that "Occupational performance consists of the 'doing' of occupation; whereas occupational form concerns the context of the doing" (1997a, p. 6). In the second edition, the concept of occupational form was explicitly presented as involving the interaction between person and environment, consistent with the ecological understanding characteristic of occupational therapy models at the time.

Another feature of the second edition was a focus on well-being and the importance of occupational performance to self-identity and a sense of fulfillment. People derive meaning and purpose from occupational performance. As Christiansen and Baum (1997b) explained, "over time, these meaningful experiences permit people to develop an understanding of who they are and what their place is in the world" (p. 48). This focus on self-identity, combined with the detailed explication of personal factors such as motivation, values, and meaning, emphasizes the biopsychosocial influence on occupational therapy. While a biomedical perspective centered on health and ill health from impairment, a biopsychosocial approach extended its concern beyond health to well being.

In the third edition of the model, person and environment are presented as separate entities that touch but are connected by two smaller circles that overlie a portion of both. These circles are occupation and performance, and they combine to create occupational performance and participation. Aligning with other editions of occupational therapy models at the time, the PEOP model acknowledged that people's ability to participate in the worlds in which they lived was important. This edition distinguished between factors intrinsic to the person, such as neurobehavioral, physiological, cognitive, psychological, emotional, and spiritual factors, and extrinsic factors, including built, natural, and cultural environments; societal factors; social interactions; and social and economic systems. These can support, enable, and restrict performance. The third edition also expanded the notion of client to include individuals, organizations, and communities.

SUMMARY

The fourth edition of the PEOP model of practice, originally created by Charles Christiansen and Carolyn Baum, presents the focus of occupational therapy as occupational performance, participation, and well-being. As an example of an ecological model, it provides guidance for practice by focusing on the transactive relationship among occupation, person, and environment, as well as emphasizing the importance of understanding the client's narrative. It emphasizes collaboration, client centeredness, and the importance of evidence to occupational therapy practice.

MEMORY AID

See Box 4.3.

BOX 4.3 ■ Person-Environment-Occupation-Performance (PEOP) Model Memory Aid

The Narrative

Occupational Profile and Client Goals

- Is this a personal narrative, an organizational narrative, or a population narrative?
- What do these people want or need to do in their daily lives and can these tasks, occupations, and roles be done successfully by these people in the current context?
- What roles (social responsibilities and privileges) do these people have and want to or intend to continue with?
- What occupations have meaning for these people and how would it affect their roles if they were unable to perform them?
- What are their past experiences and how are they shaping the present?
- What are the client's goals?

Match with occupational therapy

- Which goals can be worked on in occupational therapy?
- Are referrals required?

Person factors and environmental factors

- What person factors affect their capability to perform specific occupations in context?
- What environmental factors affect their capacity to perform specific occupations in context?
- How do these factors support, enable, or restrict the performance of activities, tasks, and roles?
- With reference to the following checklist, complete the continua of the assessment/evaluation section of the PEOP occupational therapy process.

Checklist

Person factors

- Physiological characteristics: strength, endurance, flexibility, activity levels, dress, sleep, nutrition, and health
- Cognitive dimensions: organization, reasoning, attention, awareness, executive function, and memory
- Sensory/perceptual characteristics: somatosensory, olfactory, gustatory, visual, auditory, proprioceptive, and tactile
- Motor factors: motor control, motor planning, motor learning, and postural control
- Psychological factors: emotional state (affect), self-esteem, sense of identity, self-efficacy, and theory of mind (social awareness)
- Spiritual dimensions: beliefs and practices that shape personal meaning

Environmental factors

- Social determinants of health: social support (emotional, practical, instrumental, informational) and social capital (interpersonal relationships, social receptivity, laws, policies)
- Cultural environment: values, beliefs, customs, and expectations regarding use of time
- Physical and natural environments: physical properties, tools, geography, terrain, climate, and air quality
- Assistive technology: personal technology and design, and digital technology

Intervention and Outcomes

What intervention approaches will help to achieve meaningful outcomes for this client? For each goal, assign an intervention approach from the following list:

- Create-promote
- Establish-restore
- Maintain-habilitate
- Modify-compensate
- Prevent
- Educate
- Consult
- Advocate

What will indicate that goals have been achieved?

MAJOR WORKS

Baum C, Bass J, Christiansen C. The Person-Environment-Occupation-Performance model. In: Duncan EAS, ed. *Foundations for Practice in Occupational Therapy*. 6th ed. Elsevier; 2020:87–95.

Baum C, Christiansen C. Person-Environment-Occupation-Performance: an occupation-based framework for practice. In: Christiansen CH, Baum CM, Bass-Haugen J, eds. *Occupational Therapy: Performance, Participation, and Well-Being*. 3rd ed. Slack; 2005:243–259.

Baum C, Christiansen C, Bass J. The Person-Environment-Occupation-Performance model. In: Christiansen CH, Baum CM, Bass J, eds. *Occupational Therapy: Performance, Participation, and Well-Being*. 3rd ed. Slack; 2015:243–259.

Christiansen C. Occupational therapy: intervention for life performance. In: Christiansen C, Baum C, eds. *Occupational Therapy: Overcoming Human Performance Deficits*. Slack; 1991:3–43.

Christiansen C, Baum C. Understanding occupation: definitions and concepts. In: Christiansen C, Baum C, eds. *Occupational Therapy: Enabling Function and Well-Being*. 2nd ed. Slack; 1997a:3–25.

Christiansen C, Baum C. Person-Environment-Occupational Performance: a conceptual model for practice. In: Christiansen C, Baum C, eds. *Occupational Therapy: Enabling Function and Well-Being*. 2nd ed. Slack; 1997b:47–70.

Conclusion

In this chapter we reviewed three models of practice that are often referred to as ecological models because of the particular emphasis they place on the environment. During the 1990s, there was acknowledgement in occupational therapy that the same level of attention which had been paid to the person had not been given to the environment. The first two models presented in this chapter, PEO and EHP, were developed in the 1990s and provide excellent examples of recognition that people perform occupations in specific contexts. The third model, PEOP, spans a longer period of development, with each edition being firmly situated within this ecological approach.

These ecological models of occupational therapy have been important influences in shaping the profession's understanding of occupation. The importance of the environment as central to occupation and its performance has become well accepted in the broader occupational therapy discourse. In addition, occupational therapy's emphasis on client centeredness also has its roots in this ecological tradition. This is the second of two chapters that illustrate fundamental concepts that pervade occupational therapy models. In the chapters that follow we explore five approaches that illustrate further development in occupational therapy theory and practice.

References

American Occupational Therapy Association (AOTA). Occupational therapy practice framework: domain and process. *Am J Occup Ther*. 2002 Nov-Dec;56(6):609–639.

AOTA. *Occupational Therapy Practice Framework: Domain and Process*. 3rd ed. *Am J Occup Ther*. 2014; 68:Suppl 1.

AOTA. *Occupational Therapy Practice Framework: Domain and Process*. 4th ed. *Am J Occup Ther*. 2020;74:Suppl 2.

Baum C, Bass J, Christiansen C. The Person-Environment-Occupation-Performance model. In: Duncan EAS, ed. *Foundations for Practice in Occupational Therapy*. 6th ed. Elsevier; 2020:87–95.

Baum C, Christiansen C. Person-Environment-Occupation-Performance: an occupation-based framework for practice. In: Christiansen CH, Baum CM, Bass-Haugen J, eds. *Occupational Therapy: Performance, Participation, and Well-Being*. 3rd ed. Slack; 2005:243–259.

Baum C, Christiansen C, Bass J. The Person-Environment-Occupation-Performance model. In: Christiansen CH, Baum CM, Bass JD, eds. *Occupational Therapy: Performance, Participation, and Well-Being*. 4th ed. Slack; 2015:49–55.

Bronfenbrenner U. *The Ecology of Human Development: Experiments by Nature and Design*. Harvard University Press; 1979.

Brown CE. Ecological models in occupational therapy. In: Boyt Schell BA, Gillen G, Scaffa M, eds. *Willard & Spackman's Occupational Therapy*. 13th ed. Lippincott Williams & Wilkins; 2019:622–632.

Bruner J. *Acts of Meaning*. Harvard University Press; 1989.

Christiansen C, Baum C. *Occupational Therapy: Overcoming Human Performance Deficits*. Slack; 1991.

Christiansen C, Baum C. Understanding occupation: definitions and concepts. In: Christiansen C, Baum C, eds. *Occupational Therapy: Enabling Function and Well-Being*. 2nd ed. Slack; 1997a:3–25.

Christiansen C, Baum C. Person-Environment-Occupational Performance: a conceptual model for practice. In: Christiansen C, Baum C, eds. *Occupational Therapy: Enabling Function and Well-Being*. 2nd ed. Slack; 1997b:47–70.

Christiansen CH, Baum CM, Bass JD. *Occupational Therapy: Performance, Participation, and Well-Being*. 4th ed. Slack; 2015.

Csikszentmihalyi M. *Flow: The Psychology of Optimal Experience*. Harper & Row; 1990.

Dunn W. Ecology of Human Performance model. In: Dunbar SB, ed. *Occupational Therapy Models for Intervention with Children and Families*. Slack; 2007:127–155.

Dunn W, Brown C, McGuigan A. The ecology of human performance: a framework for considering the effect of context. *Am J Occup Ther*. 1994 Jul;48(7):595–607. doi:10.5014/ajot.48.7.595

Dunn W, Brown C, Youngstrom MJ. Ecological model of occupation. In: Kramer P, Hinojosa J, Royeen CB, eds. *Perspectives in Human Occupation: Participation in Life*. Lippincott Williams & Wilkins; 2003:222–263.

Gibson JJ. *An Ecological Approach to Visual Perception*. Erlbaum; 1986.

Law M, Cooper B, Strong S, Stewart D, Rigby P, Letts L. The Person-Environment-Occupation model: a transactive approach to occupational performance. *Can J Occup Ther*. 1996 Apr;63(1):9–23. doi:10.1177/000841749606300103

Lawton MP. Competence, environmental press, and the adaption of older people. In: Lawton MP, Windley PG, Byerts TO, eds. *Aging and the Environment*. Springer; 1982:33–59.

Murray HA. *Explorations in Personality*. Oxford; 1938.

Nelson D. Occupation: form and performance. *Am J Occup Ther*. 1988 Oct;42(10):633–641. doi:10.5014/ajot.42.10.633

Reed K. An annotated history of the concepts used in occupational therapy. In: Christiansen CH, Baum CM, Bass-Haugen J, eds. *Occupational Therapy: Performance, Participation, and Well-Being*. 3rd ed. Slack; 2005:567–626.

Smith Roley S, DeLany JV, Barrows CJ, et al.; American Occupational Therapy Association Commission on Practice. Occupational therapy practice framework: domain & practice, 2nd edition. *Am J Occup Ther*. 2008 Nov-Dec;62(6):625–683. doi:10.5014/ajot.62.6.625

Occupational Therapy Practice Framework (OTPF) and Occupational Therapy Intervention Process Model (OTIPM)

CHAPTER CONTENTS

Occupational Therapy Practice Framework, Fourth Edition (OTPF-4) **88**
Major Concepts and Definitions of Terms 88
Domain 88
Process 91
Historical Description of the Framework's
 Development 96
Summary 97
Memory Aid 97
Major Works 98

Occupational Therapy Intervention Process Model (OTIPM) **99**

Major Concepts and Definitions of Terms 99
Transactional Model of Occupation 100
True Top-Down Reasoning 102
OTIPM: An Intervention Process Model 104
Historical Description of the Model's
 Development 108
Summary 109
Memory Aid 110
Major Works 110

Conclusion **111**

References **111**

In this chapter we discuss a framework and a process model that were developed in the United States. First we cover the fourth edition of the Occupational Therapy Practice Framework: Domain and Process (OTPF-4), which was developed by the American Occupational Therapy Association (AOTA) and represents the organization's official position. Then we describe the Occupational Therapy Intervention Process Model (OTIPM) and its conceptual model, the Transactional Model of Occupation. Both the OTPF-4 and the OTIPM outline the process of occupational therapy, along with a concern for practice aligning with occupational therapy's core concern. The OTPF-4 refers to this core concern using the term *domain of occupational therapy* and emphasizes that occupational therapy practitioners should work within their scope of practice and should only employ interventions that use purposeful and occupation-based approaches. The OTIPM advocates for an authentic occupational therapy practice that honors the power of occupation and enables occupational therapists to take pride in their unique professional identity. Both the framework and the model provide detailed outlines of an occupational therapy process that involves understanding the client's values, priorities, and goals relating to occupation; undertaking an evaluation process; devising appropriate interventions; and evaluating outcomes.

Occupational Therapy Practice Framework, Fourth Edition (OTPF-4)

The OTPF is an official document of the AOTA and is currently in its fourth edition (OTPF-4). The first edition of this document was "developed to articulate occupational therapy's distinct perspective and contribution to promoting the health and participation of persons, groups, and populations through engagement in occupation" (AOTA 2020, p. 2). The OTPF-4 aims to provide a structure on which to build a common understanding of the foundational concepts of occupational therapy. It is designed to be used with other knowledge and evidence that relate to the profession's practice and is appropriate to clients. It conceptualizes clients as persons, groups, and populations.

MAJOR CONCEPTS AND DEFINITIONS OF TERMS

The OTPF-4 has two major sections: the domain and the process (see Fig. 5.1). The *domain* outlines the scope of occupational therapy expertise and body of knowledge. The *process* describes the actions practitioners undertake when providing client-centered services that promote occupational engagement. Because occupational therapists understand engagement and participation in daily life in a holistic way, together the domain and the process guide occupational therapists in their work of supporting and promoting clients' participation in daily living. The OTPF-4 conceptualizes the domain and process of occupational therapy as constantly interacting in a transactional relationship for the goal of "achieving health, well-being, and participation in life through engagement in occupation" (AOTA 2020, p. 5). The distinct knowledge, skills, and qualities possessed by occupational therapists facilitate this transactional relationship and contribute to the success of occupational therapy. The OTPF-4 presents the following non-hierarchical and mutually influencing cornerstones on which occupational therapy depends and which distinguish it from other professions:

- Core values and beliefs rooted in occupation
- Knowledge of and expertise in the therapeutic use of occupation
- Professional behaviors and dispositions
- Therapeutic use of self (p. 6)

DOMAIN

The OTPF-4 outlines five aspects of the occupational therapy domain that are of equal value and exist in a dynamic interrelatedness: (1) occupations, (2) contexts, (3) performance patterns, (4) performance skills, and (5) client factors. For each aspect of the occupational therapy domain, tables are included in the OTPF-4 that provide detailed definitions, explanations, and examples. We refer readers to these tables and have not attempted to reproduce them in this chapter.

The first aspect of the occupational therapy domain is *occupations*. For occupations, the OTPF-4 used the following definition from the World Federation of Occupational Therapists (WFOT) website: "in occupational therapy, *occupations* refer to the everyday activities that people do as individuals, in families, and with communities to occupy time and bring meaning and purpose to life. Occupations include things people need to, want to and are expected to do" (WFOT 2023). The OTPF-4 distinguishes between occupation and activity by saying that occupation is personalized and meaningful whereas activity is objective and not specific to clients and their context. Both can be used as interventions. For example, the activity of chopping vegetables could be used to improve motor skills for the occupation of preparing a favorite meal. Engagement in occupation shapes a client's health, identity, and sense of competence and is considered both the means and the end of the occupational therapy process. Occupations are meaningful, purposeful, and useful to clients, and can occur over time. Some can be observed by others, and some remain private to the person engaged in them.

The OTPF-4 identifies nine broad categories of occupations: (1) activities of daily living (ADLs), (2) instrumental activities of daily living (IADLs), (3) health management, (4) rest and sleep, (5) education, (6) work, (7) play, (8) leisure, and (9) social participation. Examples of specific occupations in the category of IADLs are grocery shopping and money management (see the tables in the OTPF-4 document for detailed lists of specific occupations within each category relevant to persons, groups, and populations). While specific occupations are often linked to certain categories, the OTPF-4 acknowledges that categorization of occupations is not simple, and that clients' categorizations of specific occupations will vary widely depending on their needs, interests, and contexts, as well as cultural and sociopolitical factors.

The second aspect of the occupational therapy domain is *contexts*. The OTPF-4 defines context broadly as "the environmental and personal factors specific to each client (person, group, population) that influence engagement and participation in occupations" (p. 9). Environmental factors can be physical, social, and attitudinal and can have positive or negative effects on occupational engagement. The environmental factors listed in the OTPF-4 are (p. 10):

- Natural environment and human-made changes to the environment, including characteristics of human populations and the effect of engagement in human occupation on the sustainability of the natural environment
- Products and technology
- Support and relationships, including people and animals "that provide practical physical or emotional support, nurturing, protection, assistance, [and] connection to other persons"
- Attitudes of people other than the client
- Services, systems, and policies

Personal factors are "unique features of a person that are not part of a health condition or health state and that constitute the particular background of the person's life and living (p. 10). These are not conceptualized as positive or negative but are simply descriptive. They include beliefs, expectations, and customs a person has internalized from their cultural group as well as demographic factors. The personal factors listed in the OTPF-4 (pp. 10–11) are:

- Chronological age
- Sexual orientation
- Gender identity
- Race and ethnicity
- Cultural identification and attitudes
- Social background, social status, and socioeconomic status
- Upbringing and life experiences
- Habits, and past and current behavioral patterns
- Psychological aspects, temperament, unique character traits, and coping styles
- Education
- Profession and professional identity
- Lifestyle
- Health conditions and fitness status that are not the focus of the occupational therapy encounter

Because contextual barriers can impede people's ability to engage in occupation, occupational justice is a core concern for occupational therapy. The OTPF-4 uses the following definition of occupational justice from Nilsson and Townsend (2010): "a justice that recognizes occupational rights to inclusive participation in everyday occupations for all persons in society, regardless of age, ability, gender, social class, or other differences" (p. 58). Occupational justice is concerned with fairness and equity and with any contextual barriers to participation. Occupational injustice occurs where full occupational engagement and participation in society and people's communities is impeded by contextual factors (both environmental and personal). For example, although disabled children might be supported to engage in academic pursuits, if they have limited opportunities to engage in school life through sport, music, and social activities they are unable to participate fully. As stated in the OTPF-4, occupational therapists know that "for individuals to truly achieve full participation, meaning, and purpose, they must not only function but also engage comfortably within their own distinct combination of contexts (both environmental factors and personal factors)" (p. 11). Occupational justice involves the promotion of and access to full participation.

The third aspect of the occupational therapy domain is *performance patterns*. These are defined as "the acquired habits, routines, roles, and rituals used in the process of engaging consistently in occupations" (p. 12). Through performance patterns, people establish lifestyles and create occupational balance in their lives. Time is a central feature of performance patterns. When the performance of occupation is repeated over time it becomes a pattern of performance. *Habits* develop when performance is repeated in the same way each time. Habitual performance is automatic, reducing cognitive load and freeing up conscious attention. Habits can be healthy or unhealthy, such as daily exercise compared with regular smoking, and can be efficient or inefficient. *Routines* occur when regular sequences of occupations are established. These sequences can occur at varying intervals, such as daily, weekly, and monthly, and they can be conducted individually or with others. For example, a parent and child might engage in a nightly routine together that involves brushing teeth, dressing for bed, reading a story, and then turning off the light. Habits and routines can have positive or negative effects on a person's life and can promote or damage health. *Roles* provide structure to the ways people participate in society. Roles carry social expectations that are shaped by culture and context. Sociocultural expectations often contribute to the availability and accessibility of roles for certain people. For example, women often fulfill caring roles due to cultural expectations relating to gender, and disabled people may have difficulty obtaining paid work because of ablest societal assumptions. The roles people undertake have implications for their occupational identity because they provide social status, and people's occupational history and desires for the future will influence how they think and feel about themselves. Roles are often associated with specific activities and occupations, so they powerfully structure what people do. The final feature of performance patterns is *rituals*. These are "symbolic interactions with spiritual, cultural, or social meaning" (p. 13). People engage in certain occupations because of the meaning those occupations have for them. Rituals might be associated with a particular time of the year, week, or day and can be carried out individually or with others. They often reinforce identity, values, beliefs, and a sense of belonging to a community. (For a more in-depth discussion of habits, routines, and roles, see Chapter 6.)

The fourth aspect of the occupational therapy domain is *performance skills*. Performance skills are "observable, goal-directed actions" (p. 13). They are individual actions and are observed and analyzed for all client populations during actual performance in natural contexts. In the OTPF-4, they are categorized as motor skills, process skills, and social interaction skills with the following descriptions:

- "*Motor skills* refer to how effectively a person moves self or interacts with objects, including positioning the body, obtaining and holding objects, moving self and objects, and sustaining performance.
- *Process skills* refer to how effectively a person organizes objects, time, and space, including sustaining performance, applying knowledge, organizing timing, organizing space and objects, and adapting performance.
- *Social interactions skills* refer to how effectively a person uses both verbal and non-verbal skills to communicate, including initiating and terminating, producing, physically supporting, shaping content of, maintaining flow of, verbally supporting, and adapting social interaction" (p. 13).

Examples of motor skills include bending, grasping, manipulating, and coordinating and calibrating movements. Examples of process skills include initiating and sequencing steps, and planning and organizing. Examples of social interaction skills include using facial expressions, gesturing, taking turns, and responding.

The fifth aspect of the occupational therapy domain is *client factors*. While performance skills are observable actions, client factors are internal to people and are influenced by "the presence or absence of illness, disease, deprivation and disability, as well as by life stages and experiences" (p. 15). Specific client factors listed in the OTPF-4 are values, beliefs, and spirituality, which influence motivation for occupational engagement and give meaning to life, as well as body functions and structures, such as physiological functions and anatomical structures. Client factors influence and are influenced by the other four aspects of the occupational therapy domain, and it is important to remember that limitations in body functions and structures alone do not determine the quality and success of occupational performance. For example, altering the context and/or the way people conduct occupation can improve the success of occupational performance and enhance occupational participation without necessarily altering body functions and structures.

These five aspects comprise the domain of occupational therapy, which centers on occupational engagement and performance. By addressing all five aspects of the domain, occupational therapists can ensure that they are addressing the full scope of occupational therapy. The five aspects of occupational therapy must be understood as intimately connected and mutually influencing, contributing to a fluid whole that is constantly changing as people conduct their daily lives. While the domain guides occupational therapists in their scope of practice, the process outlines how occupational therapists work collaboratively with their clients.

PROCESS

The occupational therapy *process* describes the client-centered delivery of services and has three parts: "1) evaluation and 2) intervention to achieve 3) targeted outcomes" (p. 17) (refer to Fig. 5.1).

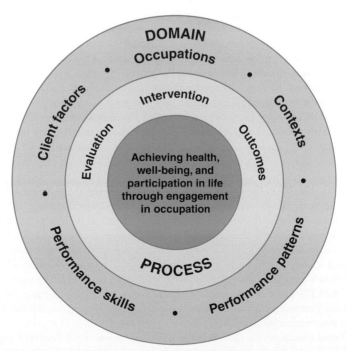

Fig. 5.1 Occupational therapy domain and process. (From AOTA. Occupational therapy practice framework: domain and process—fourth edition. *Am J Occup Ther.* 2020 Aug 1;74(Supplement_2):5. doi:10.5014/ajot.2020. 74S2001)

Throughout this process and from a perspective based on the cornerstones of occupational therapy, occupational therapists engage in clinical and professional reasoning, analyze occupations and activities, and collaborate with clients. Their unique perspective involves:

- Using occupation to promote health, well-being, and participation in life
- Understanding occupational participation as resulting from the mutual influence of clients, their contexts, and the occupations in which they engage
- Basing their choices on the knowledge, theories, and skills from which the profession draws

The OTPF-4 presents occupational therapy service provision as a dynamic and fluid process that remains focused on targeted outcomes. This requires constantly adapting and changing the methods used as circumstances change and understandings of the client's situation evolve. Occupational therapists can provide direct and indirect services. Direct services are delivered collaboratively and may be offered face-to-face or remotely through telehealth. Direct services can be at the person level, such as inpatient rehabilitation and working with a schoolchild while collaborating with their teacher; at the group level, such as a cooking group at a skilled nursing facility; and at the population level, such as large-scale healthy living or driver training initiatives in the community. Indirect services might involve advocating on behalf of clients to other entities such as organizations, multidisciplinary teams, teachers, and government and community agencies. Occupational therapists also practice at organizational and systems levels because these are often the mechanisms through which occupational needs can be met. Examples of such interventions include the development of a falls prevention program for skilled nursing facilities, recommendations for ergonomic changes that decrease the risk of injury at a specific workplace, and advocating for changes to building standards and repair of footpaths.

The three core skills discussed in the OTPF-4 as used throughout the occupational therapy process are (1) occupational analysis and activity analysis, (2) therapeutic use of self, and (3) clinical and professional reasoning. According to the OTPF-4, *occupational analysis* is contextual and specific and requires an understanding of the client's circumstances and "the specific occupations the client wants or needs to do in the actual context in which these occupations are performed" (p. 20). In contrast, *activity analysis* is decontextualized and generic, laying out the typical demands of the activity within a particular culture. Of these two, occupational analysis is unique to occupational therapy. Occupational and activity analyses can reveal the performance patterns, performance skills, and client factors required for performance.

The *therapeutic use of self* involves developing and managing relationships with clients "by using professional reasoning, empathy, and a client-centered, collaborative approach to service delivery" (p. 20). Using their clinical reasoning, occupational therapists assist clients to process their experiences and develop a sense of meaning and hope. Through empathy, they develop an emotional connection with their clients that allows for open communication and builds trust. Using a client-centered, collaborative approach enables power sharing and acknowledges the contribution of both clients and practitioners to the occupational therapy encounter. Clients contribute knowledge of their lives and circumstances as well as their hopes and dreams. Occupational therapists contribute their knowledge of the power of occupation to influence health, well-being, and participation in life. Through their therapeutic use of self, they create relationships in which clients can feel safe and free to express their true identities. They help clients understand their experiences and collaboratively develop a vision for occupational therapy intervention. As the OTPF-4 states, "practitioners and clients, together with caregivers, family members, community members, and other stakeholders (as appropriate), identify and prioritize the focus of the intervention plan" (p. 20).

Occupational therapists use clinical and professional reasoning throughout the occupational therapy process to identify the meanings of and skills required for the client's occupational performance in their context. For the concept of clinical and professional reasoning, the OTPF-4 uses the term *professional reasoning* to encompass the broad settings in which occupational therapists work. Occupational therapists use professional reasoning to develop a rich understanding of how the interrelated aspects of the domain are contributing to occupational performance. They use occupational therapy's knowledge base of models, theories, and evidence to guide their professional reasoning when making decisions about evaluation and intervention. They also use their professional reasoning when considering how to encourage their client's participation in occupations.

Turning now to the occupational therapy process, the first step is *evaluation*. This involves collecting information that contributes to an in-depth understanding of the client's occupational needs and enables the identification of targeted outcomes. Evaluation consists of the development of an occupational profile and the analysis of occupational performance, after which a synthesis of the evaluation process is undertaken. While the components of evaluation are discussed separately, the client's needs, practice setting, and model of practice or frame of reference being used will all influence exactly how information is collected and in what order. The OTPF-4 also states that the process of evaluation for groups and populations mirrors that for individuals. In some settings, a screening or consultation process is undertaken to determine whether a full occupational therapy evaluation is required. The screening processes may result in a brief occupational profile or recommendations for a full evaluation.

The *occupational profile* contributes to an understanding of the client's circumstances and their perspectives on life. It includes the client's "occupational history and experiences, patterns of daily living, interests, values, needs, and relevant contexts" (p. 21). It explores what is meaningful in the client's daily life and provides background history that could shed light on current occupational issues. The goal of developing an occupational profile is to identify outcomes that are meaningful and important to clients. Only clients can determine what is most meaningful in their lives and identify their priorities. Therefore, by respecting and valuing client input, occupational therapists can create situations in which clients are empowered to participate and interventions can be more effectively chosen. Information for the occupational profile is collected early in the occupational therapy process, and the profile can then be refined as greater understanding develops over time. Information can be gathered at one time or over a longer period using formal and informal techniques, and can also be obtained from clients and significant others as appropriate. The type of information gathered for the occupational profile includes:

- The reason the client is seeking occupational therapy services
- The client's priorities and targeted outcomes relating to their health, well-being, and occupational participation
- The client's occupational history, values, beliefs, and interests
- The client's perceptions of occupations in which they experience success and barriers that inhibit their success in other occupations
- The client's identification of aspects of their contexts (environmental and personal factors) and of their performance patterns that promote or impede occupational engagement
- The client's current patterns of occupational engagement and how these have changed over time
- The client's perceptions of client factors (i.e., those relating to the health condition, such as pain and active symptoms) that affect their occupational performance and engagement

Once profile information has been collected, occupational therapists hypothesize about possible reasons for the issues and concerns identified. Potential reasons might relate to performance skills, performance patterns, client factors, and context. Occupational profile information is used to individualize approaches to evaluation and intervention planning and implementation.

Regarding *analysis of occupational performance*, the OTPF-4 states that "*occupational performance* is the accomplishment of the selected occupation resulting from the dynamic transaction among the client, their contexts, and the occupation. In the *analysis of occupational performance*, the practitioner identifies the client's ability to effectively complete desired occupations" (p. 22, italics in original). The process of undertaking an analysis of occupational performance commences with determining the occupations and contexts that need to be addressed. Information for this primarily comes from the occupational profile, which has identified meaningful and important outcomes. Occupational and activity analyses are conducted on relevant occupations and contexts to identify the demands on the client. Specific assessments are then selected to measure the effect on occupational performance of (1) the client's performance or performance deficits while completing these occupations, especially their performance skills and performance patterns; (2) client factors; and (3) the client's contexts. Formal and informal assessment tools are used to analyze, measure, and investigate the factors that promote or hinder occupational performance. The OTPF-4 makes it clear that standardized assessments are preferred when available because these provide objective information. However, multiple methods of information gathering are generally used during evaluation, including observation of occupational performance, interviews, and discussions. Trustworthy information from valid and reliable assessments can evidence the need for occupational therapy services and provide a baseline with which to compare the results of occupational therapy intervention.

Once information has been collected and analysis undertaken, a synthesis of the evaluation process is created. This synthesis can include:

- Identifying the client's values and priorities regarding occupational performance
- Interpreting assessment results to determine facilitators of and barriers to performance of these occupations
- Developing and refining hypotheses regarding strengths and weaknesses in the client's occupational performance
- Identifying resources available to support the intervention process
- Determining targeted outcomes of the intervention process and identifying goals collaboratively with the client to address these outcomes
- Selecting outcome measures that are commensurate with the client's values and beliefs and the practitioner's theoretical model of practice

Intervention is the second step in the occupational therapy process. Services are provided by occupational therapists and aim to promote occupational engagement and enhance health and well-being through achievement of targeted outcomes. Service provision must be consistent with the service delivery model and be undertaken in collaboration with clients. Occupational therapists combine the information they have gathered from and about the client with theoretical principles to select and provide appropriate occupation-based interventions. The OTPF-4 identifies the following common aims of intervention: (1) create or promote, (2) establish or restore, (3) maintain, (4) modify, and (5) prevent. It categorizes the types of interventions an occupational therapist might use as (1) occupations and activities, (2) interventions to support occupations, (3) education and training, (4) advocacy, (5) group interventions, and (6) virtual interventions. When carrying out interventions, occupational therapists are expected to comply with ethical codes and standards.

Interventions vary according to the nature of the client (person, group, or population) and the service delivery context. Individual clients might be referred to as patients or students and organizational clients might be called consumers or members. Other people involved indirectly might be, for example, parents, teachers, caregivers, employers, and spouses. The OTPF-4 states that "occupational therapy practitioners work with a wide variety of populations experiencing difficulty in accessing and engaging in healthy occupations because of factors such as poverty, homelessness, displacement, and discrimination" (p. 24) and gives the example of refugees and asylum seekers. When services are provided to groups and populations, they could involve direct service provision or consultation. They might include recommendations for change management for an organization, or strategies for health promotion, prevention, and screening of populations for governments.

In the OTPF-4, intervention is divided into three components: (1) intervention plan, (2) intervention implementation, and (3) intervention review. Throughout the intervention process, occupational therapy practitioners use their professional reasoning, which is shaped by "theory, practice models, frames of reference, and research evidence on interventions" (p. 25) as well as their knowledge of the client. Occupational therapists begin the intervention process by creating an intervention plan. This plan guides the actions of occupational therapists by outlining the intervention types and approaches that will be used. The intervention plan is developed in collaboration with clients (or their proxies) and considers their health and well-being, values and priorities, and occupational needs, as well as the practitioner's evaluation of the interaction among client factors, contexts, occupation and activity demands, client performance skills and performance patterns, and best available evidence. The intervention plan outlines the goals of therapy and the intervention approaches and methods that will be used. It also considers potential discharge needs and referrals to other professionals that might be required. Once the intervention plan has been created, intervention implementation is undertaken and may include:

- "therapeutic use of occupations and activities
- interventions to support occupations
- education
- training
- advocacy
- self-advocacy
- group interventions
- virtual interventions" (p. 25)

Occupational therapists attend closely to the client's responses and continually adapt the intervention, evaluate, and reevaluate throughout. Thus the process of intervention review commences while intervention implementation is being undertaken. This includes determining whether occupational therapy services should be continued or discontinued and whether referrals should be made to other professionals.

Outcomes is the third part of the occupational therapy process, and their consideration is undertaken throughout the process. Identifying potential outcomes is the purpose of evaluation, and working to achieve outcomes is the purpose of intervention. The OTPF-4 summarizes the targeted outcomes of occupational therapy as occupational performance, prevention, health and wellness, quality of life, participation, role competence, well-being, and occupational justice. The outcomes that are targeted may change throughout the occupational therapy process, as circumstances and client factors change and as understanding of the client's occupational needs changes. Outcomes are measured against the baseline measurements obtained during evaluation. Objective measurements are used to determine improvement in occupational performance. Some settings use patient-reported outcomes (PROs) to obtain the client's subjective responses. "PROs can be used as subjective measures of improved outlook, confidence, hope, playfulness, self-efficacy, sustainability of valued occupations, pain reduction, resilience, and well-being" (p. 27). Outcomes can also be obtained from caregivers, particularly in relation to indicators such as quality of life of both clients and caregivers. The OTPF-4 also provides examples of outcomes for groups, such as improved social interaction, expanded social support, and increased self-awareness from peer interaction, as well as outcomes for populations, such as improved health literacy and accessibility of public spaces and resources, increased community integration, and expanded access to services.

A final consideration in the occupational therapy process is transition and discontinuation of occupational therapy service. Planning may be required when a transition from one service to another is needed. For example, this might require referral or preparation of the client for the new service. Discontinuation of the current service may also require planning. For example, certain equipment might be needed prior to discharge from a hospital, or a person might require psychological preparation before discontinuing participation in a group.

In summary, the OTPF-4 provides a framework for achieving health, well-being, and participation in life through engagement in occupation. It outlines both the domain and the process

BOX 5.1 ■ OTPF-4 Case Illustration

Alex is a final-year occupational therapy student undertaking a placement in a community psychiatric facility. One client assigned to him is Chris, who is 45 years old, identifies as gender nonbinary, and was diagnosed with schizophrenia 20 years ago. Chris would like to participate in a work integration program, but their family has never allowed them to work. Alex used the OTPF-4 to guide the assessment process and develop a comprehensive understanding of their situation.

In the initial interview, Alex explored Chris's personal factors and found that they are single, live with their sister, and do not have children. They come from a high economic background. Chris finished high school but did not continue formal education after that. They have never worked and are financially supported by their family. In relation to their performance patterns, Chris's main habits and routines involve waking up early, spending 30 minutes exercising, and after taking a shower, participating in gardening activities with their sister. Chris described their principal roles as being sibling, offspring, and dog owner. Alex conducted some standardized assessments and interviews, and Chris completed some self-report questionnaires. The results informed Alex about Chris's performance skills. In terms of their motor skills, their gross motor coordination is appropriate to their age, but the weight they have gained as a side effect of their antipsychotic medications affects their ability to move around. For example, they struggle to get up from chairs, and they have pain in their knees when they walk to the shops, walk the dog, and climb stairs. Cognitively, Chris has difficulties with short-term memory and a reduced attention span. Their social skills are limited because sometimes they express their feelings and ideas without considering others and suffer from mood swings caused by paranoid ideation. They frequently say things that are offensive to other people without meaning to upset them. In terms of their process skills, Chris has difficulties sustaining and adapting their performance in most occupations and has problems with organizing time and tasks. In terms of personal factors, Chris deeply values their relationship with their sister, parents, and dog, and has a profound faith in God.

Informed by the results of the evaluation process, Alex worked collaboratively with Chris to establish an intervention plan based on their interests and priorities. Chris is highly motivated to be part of the gardening program and learn new skills with a view to being employed for the first time in their life. The intervention implementation involved training for specific gardening tasks and education about plants and irrigation, with the purpose of increasing their role competence and improving their occupational performance as a gardener. Alex taught Chris some cognitive strategies that enabled them to use their strengths to overcome the challenges related to cognition that were affecting their performance, and to achieve their goals. Alex also met with Chris's family to advocate for Chris and educate the family on the advantages of giving Chris the opportunity to be employed, explaining that people with mental illness frequently have poor access to employment and its health-promoting benefits. Alex knew that facilitating access to employment would achieve occupational justice for Chris. Following the last step of the OTPF-4 process, Alex developed a transition plan and made connections with an employment program where Chris would be able to work after finishing the intervention process.

of occupational therapy. The domain of occupational therapy refers to its scope, and the OTPF-4 discusses the domain in terms of occupations, contexts, performance patterns, performance skills, and client factors. The process of occupational therapy involves evaluation, intervention, and the identification and evaluation of targeted outcomes. Throughout the process, occupational therapists use their clinical reasoning combined with the professional knowledge base and evidence. Box 5.1 provides a case about Alex and Chris that illustrates an OTPF-4 perspective. In the section that follows, we describe the development of the OTPF-4 in its broader context as an official document of the AOTA.

HISTORICAL DESCRIPTION OF THE FRAMEWORK'S DEVELOPMENT

The OTPF-4 is part of a continual process of documenting the official position of the AOTA. This process commenced with the Occupational Therapy Product Output Reporting System and

Uniform Terminology for Reporting Occupational Therapy Services (AOTA 1979). This was followed by *Uniform Terminology for Occupational Therapy, Second Edition (UT-II)* (AOTA 1989), which described the occupational performance areas and components addressed by occupational therapists. This document aligns with the occupational performance models prevalent at the time (see Chapter 3), demonstrating the influence of a biomedical perspective. The third and final edition of *Uniform Terminology for Occupational Therapy*, known as *UT-III*, was "expanded to reflect current practice and to incorporate contextual aspects of performance" (AOTA 1994, p. 1047). These additions demonstrate the adoption of a biopsychosocial perspective.

The OTPF (AOTA 2002) was developed after a review of *UT-III* and aimed to provide a fuller description of contemporary occupational therapy. The OTPF is an evolving document and is reviewed by the AOTA Commission on Practice every five years to maintain its usefulness and identify any refinements or changes required. For this review, the Commission on Practice obtains feedback from "AOTA members, scholars, authors, practitioners, AOTA volunteer leadership and staff, and other stakeholders" (AOTA 2020, p. 3). This quinquennial review of the OTPF resulted in the OTPF-2 (AOTA 2008) and then the OTPF-3 (AOTA 2014). In the OTPF-4 (AOTA 2020), the major changes include an increased focus on groups and populations, a more explicit explanation of occupational science, a description of cornerstones of occupational therapy practice, clearer definitions of occupation and activity, changes to various definitions and categorization terms and concepts, and alterations to terminology to align more closely with the *International Classification of Functioning, Disability and Health (ICF)*. The OTPF-4 is "occupation based, client centered, contextual, and evidence based" (AOTA 2020, p. 4) and continues the founding values of occupational therapy and the founders' vision for the profession of using occupation to remediate illness and maintain health in the context of a therapeutic relationship that pays close attention to the client's circumstances, values, and goals.

SUMMARY

The OTPF-4 outlines the scope of occupational therapy expertise and body of knowledge (domain). It also identifies practitioners' actions when providing client-centered services that promote participation in daily life through occupational engagement (process). It conceptualizes the purpose of occupational therapy as "achieving health, well-being, and participation in life through engagement in occupation" (AOTA 2020, p. 5). The domain of occupational therapy has five components that exist in dynamic interrelatedness: occupations, contexts, performance patterns, performance skills, and client factors. The process of occupational therapy involves evaluation and intervention to achieve outcomes. Throughout this process, occupational therapists engage in clinical and professional reasoning, analyze occupations and activities, and collaborate with clients.

Occupational therapists conceptualize occupational engagement as resulting from a dynamic transaction among the client, their contexts, and the occupation. They have distinct knowledge, skills, and qualities, and can be distinguished from other professions by their core values and beliefs rooted in occupation, their knowledge of and expertise in the therapeutic use of occupation, their professional behaviors and dispositions, and their therapeutic use of self. The OTPF-4 provides a framework for guiding occupational therapists' reasoning and actions, supporting them to provide quality occupational therapy services. It is an official document of the AOTA and is reviewed every five years to ensure that it reflects current thinking and practice. It provides substantial and detailed tables outlining concepts and their use in practice, and readers are encouraged to access them.

MEMORY AID

See Box 5.2.

BOX 5.2 ■ OTPF Memory Aid

Evaluation

- Is a full evaluation or a screening evaluation required?
- What information do I need to collect to understand the client's circumstances and occupational needs?
- How could I collect this?
- How can I ensure that there is client input into this process?
  Create an occupational profile that highlights the client's circumstances and perspective on life.
- Why is the client seeking occupational therapy services?
- What outcomes are meaningful and important to the client?

  Consider the client's occupational history and experiences, patterns of daily living, interests, values, needs, and relevant contexts.
- What are some possible reasons for the issues and concerns identified? (e.g., performance skills, performance patterns, client factors and context)
  Undertake an analysis of occupational performance.
- What occupations and contexts need to be addressed?
- What specific methods (formal and informal assessment tools) can I use to measure the effect on occupational performance of the client's performance skills and performance patterns, client factors, and the client's context?
  Evaluation synthesis—synthesize evaluation information, considering the following:

- The client's values and priorities regarding occupational performance
- Results of assessments and reasoning regarding occupational performance
- Resources available to facilitate occupational performance
- Collaboratively determined goals and outcomes, and how they will be evaluated

Outcomes

What targeted outcomes could contribute to improving the client's health, well-being, and participation in life? (The client could be an individual, group, or population.)
- Consider occupational performance, prevention, health and wellness, quality of life, participation, role competence, well-being, and occupational justice.
- As I have collected more information and gained a more in-depth understanding of the client's circumstances, do these outcomes need to be revised and, if so, how?

Intervention

- What is expected of occupational therapy by clients and the service delivery model?
- What aims are appropriate for this client? (e.g., create or promote, establish or restore, maintain, modify, and prevent)
- What interventions might be appropriate? (e.g., occupations and activities; interventions to support occupations; education and training; advocacy; group interventions; virtual interventions)

Final Outcomes

- Have targeted outcomes been achieved? What planning is required for discontinuation of service?

MAJOR WORKS

AOTA. Occupational therapy practice framework: domain and process—fourth edition. *Am J Occup Ther.* 2020 Aug 1;74(Supplement_2):7412410010p1–7412410010p87. doi:10.5014/ajot.2020.74S2001

Occupational Therapy Intervention Process Model (OTIPM)

The OTIPM was developed by Anne Fisher and its most recent version is published in *Powerful Practice: A Model for Authentic Occupational Therapy* (Fisher and Marterella 2019). It aims to provide an integrated, occupation-centered reasoning model that guides occupational therapists to practice in an authentic and powerful manner. By focusing on occupation, the OTIPM makes explicit the fact that occupation is the primary concern of occupational therapists and provides a rationale for how they see themselves (as *occupational* therapists) and what they do (address the *occupational* concerns of their clients). Occupational therapists use occupation-centered reasoning, which highlights their unique philosophical perspective and guides the practical implementation of occupational therapy services. This perspective conceptualizes people as occupational beings for whom occupation is vital and who face occupational challenges in their lives.

MAJOR CONCEPTS AND DEFINITIONS OF TERMS

Fisher and Marterella (2019) made it clear that the OTIPM is the primary model in the overall integrated, occupation-centered reasoning model presented in *Powerful Practice*. In discussing the OTIPM, they distinguished between process-driven and theory-driven practice, making it clear that occupational therapists using the OTIPM are engaged in process-driven practice and that the OTIPM is a process model. As Fisher and Marterella explained, process models "delineate the steps in the occupational therapy process" (p. 5) from beginning to end. The OTIPM comprises five steps that are grouped into three phases:

1. Evaluation and goal-setting phase
    1. Gather initial information
    2. Implement performance analyses
    3. Finalize evaluation
2. Intervention phase
    4. Select model(s) of practice and planning and implement intervention
3. Reevaluation phase
    5. Implement reevaluation and ascertain outcomes

Two types of theory-driven practice models are used in conjunction with the OTIPM and are presented in *Powerful Practice*. First, the Transactional Model of Occupation is presented as a conceptual model. Conceptual models make explicit the concepts and assumptions upon which practice is based. This model presents a transactional perspective of occupation, whereby occupation must be understood as part of a transactional whole in which all elements of the whole are in a state of constant transaction. As Fisher and Marterella (2019) explained, "this holistic perspective reminds occupational therapists that they cannot separate people from their situational contexts or their past, present, and future experiences, and it brings sociocultural, geopolitical, and environmental influences on occupation to the foreground" (p. 16). The Transactional Model of Occupation does not present person, environment, and occupation as separate entities that contribute to occupational performance, as has been common in occupational therapy, but as three of many elements that contribute to a holistic view of occupation (the Transactional Model of Occupation is discussed in the next section). Second, *Powerful Practice* presents four theory-driven intervention models to be used with the OTIPM: a compensatory model, an education and teaching model, an acquisitional model, and a restorative model. It also presents a mixed-models approach. These models, which are linked to the intervention phase of the process model, outline the principles and methods used for intervention and assist occupational therapists to authentically focus on occupation.

As a process model, the OTIPM provides a framework for assisting occupational therapists to reason, plan, and implement services that are occupational. Fisher and Marterella (2019) argued that process models can be more flexible and less restrictive than theory-driven approaches and can guide occupational therapists to provide inspired, high-quality occupational therapy services. The step-by-step process outlined in the OTIPM guides therapists to develop occupation-centered reasoning, in which occupational therapy's unique perspective provides the "starting point of everything occupational therapists do" (p. 3) and drives implementation of services that are occupational.

TRANSACTIONAL MODEL OF OCCUPATION

The Transactional Model of Occupation presents a transactional understanding of occupation. Fisher and Marterella (2019) acknowledged the work of Dickie and colleagues (2006) in introducing a transactional perspective of occupation to occupational science. A transactional perspective emphasizes the situatedness of occupation and conceptualizes it as "a continual response to situational elements that mutually shape each other" (p. 16). In the diagram of the model, occupation is placed in the center and is presented as having three interwoven occupational elements: occupational performance, occupational experience, and participation. Surrounding the center, and connected to occupation through multiple dotted lines, are seven situational elements: geopolitical, sociocultural, temporal, social environment, physical environment, task, and client (note that client is one of the situational elements of occupation, rather than being presented as an entity separate from occupation). In seeking to represent the complexity of the relationships among the occupational and situational elements, Fisher and Marterella stated that "to convey this complex relational idea visually, we have used a background image of a swirl to convey the idea that all of the situation elements 'swirl together' and merge with occupation to create an inextricably intertwined transactional whole" (p. 16). Thus occupation cannot be separated from its situational elements, and all aspects of the transactional whole influence and shape one another.

Fisher and Marterella (2019) discussed each occupational and situational element of the transactional whole. The first of three occupational elements, *occupational performance*, refers to the observable aspects of a person's doing. Occupational performance can be considered at a broader level and at a discrete level. The broader level refers to performance of activities and tasks. While acknowledging that activities can be categorized in many ways, Fisher and Marterella listed categories such as ADLs, leisure activities, social activities, and work activities. The broader level can also refer to the performance of specific tasks, such as dressing and eating. At the discrete level, performance skills are the smallest observable units of occupations and include abilities such as reaching and grasping. These are linked together into a chain of observable, goal-directed actions. Activity and task performances, as well as performance skills, can be observed. In contrast, the second occupational element, *occupational experience*, which refers to people's experience of occupational performance, cannot be observed. Therefore it is often elicited from clients through self-report. Clients might report their experiences verbally, or occupational therapists may observe a client's nonverbal communication through gestures such as facial expressions and body language. Regardless, occupational therapists need to work toward understanding the experiences of their clients. The third occupational element, *participation*, occurs when someone experiences personal value while engaged in an activity. Examples of personal value associated with activities include feeling that something is worthwhile and that, by doing it, one is making a difference and helping; feeling that something is necessary or that one is required, compelled, or obliged to do it; engaging in something because of having made a commitment or having a responsibility to do it; doing something because one has always done it; and feeling accepted, included, and socially connected by engaging in it. Fisher and Marterella emphasized four points about participation. First, people gain a sense of participating in society through the process of engaging in valued occupations in their communities. Second, because occupation (and therefore participation) is embedded in and inextricably connected to a constantly changing situation, each time someone participates, their participation will be different because the situation is different. Third, people can be actively engaged and participating without necessarily performing occupation. Examples of active engagement without performance include listening to music, watching sports, and talking about previous experiences. Finally, because people cannot be separated from their situational contexts, their sense of participation is always situated in a particular society.

The Transactional Model of Occupation diagram in *Powerful Practice* presents the seven situational elements as a swirling background that is in constant flux. These elements are connected to each other and to occupation through this swirl and through dotted lines. As Fisher and Marterella (2019) stated, the diagram urges "occupational therapists to keep in mind that each of these situational elements is part of a greater relational whole and inextricably intertwined with occupation and all the other situational elements... Because people cannot be separated from their situational contexts, client elements necessarily become part of the client's situational context" (p. 23). For each of the seven situational elements, the diagram provides bulleted lists that aim to serve as examples "to stimulate thinking about the breath, depth, and complexity of occupation" (p. 23), rather than as comprehensive lists. The first three situational elements—geopolitical, sociocultural, and temporal—point to the broadest aspects of occupation's situatedness. While these are important to consider, they are often neglected in occupational therapy. *Geopolitical elements* include geographic, political, economic, and historical factors. These elements remind occupational therapists that occupations vary across geographic regions and are constrained or facilitated by the policies and decisions that flow from the political and economic context. Taking a historical perspective on occupation prompts occupational therapists to consider how occupation changes over time, particularly as technology advances. *Sociocultural elements* include rules, regulations, and norms; attitudes and expectations; shared morals, beliefs, values, and customs; and ethical considerations. These all have implications for what people do, and when, where, and how they do it, as well as what they think others will expect of them. Variations in sociocultural elements across cultures are acknowledged, and occupational therapists are reminded of their ethical obligation to uphold the rights of clients, particularly their rights to privacy, to dignity of risk, and to make culturally aligned choices. *Temporal elements* include past, present, and future; patterns, sequences, and rhythms; and duration and frequency. Time is a crucial aspect of occupation. Occupational performance unfolds through a sequence of actions over time, and people's current experiences of occupation are shaped by their previous experiences and will influence their future experiences. Occupations also differ in terms of when they are done, how often, how long they last, whether they must be done using a standard procedure and in a certain order or can be done flexibly, and whether they can be done in tandem with other occupations or must be done individually.

While the geopolitical, sociocultural, and temporal elements draw occupational therapists' attention to the broadest aspects of the situational context, the social and physical environmental elements are often experienced by people more directly and are more obvious. The *social environmental element* includes other people, others' characteristics, others' personal meanings and expectations, pets and service animals, and connections and relationships. The people and animals connected to clients, whether present or not, influence their occupations and are influenced by them. These social connections might bring expectations, obligations, a sense of connectedness, purpose, and strong emotional reactions. They will influence and be influenced by what people do. The *physical environmental elements* include spaces, tangible objects, and digital environments. The physical environment is commonly considered by occupational therapists.

The last two of the situational elements in the Transactional Model of Occupation—the task and client elements—have long been considered in occupational therapy as separate entities, so thinking transactionally about these elements might be quite a challenge for occupational therapists. However, the task and client elements need to be conceptualized as just two of the seven situational elements that are in constant transaction and which will shape and be shaped by occupation. *Task elements* relate to expectations regarding occupation and include expected structure and timing; expected spaces, tools, and materials; and intended purpose or outcome. *Client elements* are features of the situational context that are internal to the client (the client could be an individual, collective, or group). These include personal factors; embodied habits, routines, rituals, and roles; attitudes, beliefs, interests, and values; occupational priorities; and body functions. To emphasize a transactional perspective on the client, Fisher and Marterella (2019) explained that, from a transactional perspective, people do not produce occupation. Instead, occupation is a response to the situational whole in which all the situational elements are in constant transaction (including the client). The client is only one of seven situational elements that combine to produce occupation. Each instance of occupational performance and people's experiences and sense of participation will be different as the swirl of situational elements creates unique situations.

TRUE TOP-DOWN REASONING

While the OTIPM is underpinned conceptually by a transactional understanding of occupation, another important foundation is the assumption that, to be properly occupation centered, occupational therapists need to use true top-down, occupation-centered reasoning. Fisher and Marterella (2019) contrasted true top-down reasoning with bottom-up and top-to-bottom-up reasoning (see Fig. 5.2). In advocating true top-down reasoning as the key to authentic occupational practice, they emphasize the degree to which these three types of reasoning differ in terms of whether they focus on occupation and include observation of actual client performance. As they explained, *bottom-up reasoning* commences with an evaluation of body functions and/or environmental factors. This leads to speculation about how these factors are impacting a client's occupational performance. This kind of reasoning is most associated with traditional occupational performance models (see Chapter 3) in which evaluation methods that do not consider people's specific life contexts are used, such as those largely focused on body functions (e.g., range of motion, muscle strength, cognition, and emotional regulation). Speculation is also undertaken regarding environmental factors that are possibly restricting occupational performance. These evaluations of body and environment are often paired with activity analyses, whereby activities are analyzed into their component parts. (As we explain later, activity analysis centers on the demands of the activity rather than observation of a person's performance of that activity.) Together they are used to speculate how these elements are impacting occupational performance. Some of the problems identified in using a bottom-up evaluation approach include the risk of planning and implementing interventions to address impairments in body functions without understanding the client's concerns regarding their occupational performance and their needs and desires for occupation and participation in society; assuming that occupation is only influenced by impairments in body functions and failing to take a holistic view of the complexity of factors that shape occupation; and not undertaking evaluation of the quality of the client's actual performance of occupation.

The *top-to-bottom-up reasoning* approach commences by exploring the client's desires and needs regarding occupation and participation and their concerns about their occupational performance. Fisher and Marterella (2019) outlined how a top-to-bottom-up approach proceeds "from the top... to the bottom... then going back up and speculating about which body functions, environmental factors, or other contextual factors are impacting the client's reported problems with occupational performance" (p. 39). One problem with the top-to-bottom-up approach is that it relies on clients' self-reported problems rather than direct observation. This does not enable occupational therapists to evaluate the quality of a client's occupational performance. A second

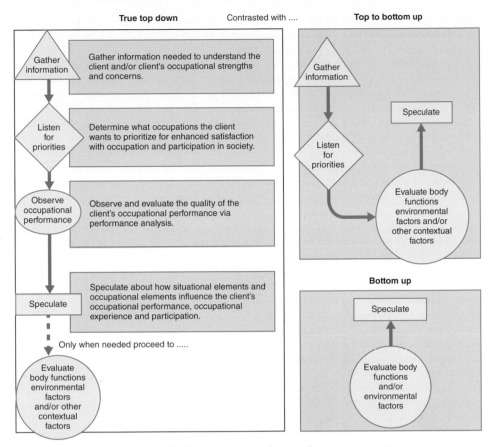

Fig. 5.2 Comparison of approaches.

problem with the top-to-bottom-up approach is that it "views occupation as being separate from or produced by people who are interacting with the environment as they perform tasks" (p. 39). They argue that a long and widely held perspective in occupational therapy is that person, environment, and occupation are separate entities that interact to facilitate or impede occupational performance and participation. In contrast, a transactional view of occupation places occupation at the center and views it holistically as an organic process comprising environmental, task, client, temporal, sociocultural, and geopolitical elements that are in constant and mutually influencing transaction.

True top-down reasoning is the approach advocated in *Powerful Practice*. It overcomes the two problems identified in relation to the top-to-bottom-up reasoning approach. First, a key step in the true top-down reasoning approach is to observe and evaluate the client's actual occupational performance. This enables occupational therapists to place occupation at the center of their practice—they can be *occupational* therapists. Body functions, environmental factors, and other contextual factors are only evaluated as needed. This helps avoid the risk of falling into the trap of becoming a specialist in body functions rather than practicing authentic occupational therapy. Second, by being guided by the Transactional Model of Occupation, the concept of occupation is transformed from a simple entity such as occupational performance to a holistic entity of mutually influencing elements. Therefore the speculative aspect of this reasoning process is not limited to body functions and environmental factors but encompasses how situational elements and occupational elements transact and *result* in occupation.

A unique feature of true top-down reasoning is observing and evaluating the quality of the client's occupational performance. Occupational therapists can observe this quality at the broader level of overall task performance as well as the more specific level of observable, goal-directed actions or performance skills. Performance analyses are used to evaluate the quality of these actions or performance skills (e.g., reaching, gripping, holding) when they work together for the performance of tasks (e.g., brushing teeth). Performance analysis is one of four types of analysis outlined in the OTIPM. Performance analysis, along with expanded task analysis and traditional task analysis, are associated with a true top-down approach because they are based on observation of the client's actual occupational performance. OTIPM uses the term *occupation-based* to refer to evaluations and interventions that are based on clients engaging in occupation. Therefore all three types of analysis are occupation based.

Performance analysis evaluates the quality of a client's occupational performance at the level of actions or performance skills. When using a true top-down approach, the first step is always to undertake performance analysis to evaluate the quality of the client's occupational performance through observation. This can be followed by *expanded task analysis*, which involves reflection on observed occupational performance. In this reflection, occupational therapists use the Transactional Model of Occupation to guide speculation on how the situational and occupational elements transact together and result in the quality of occupational performance they have observed. Both types of analysis are also occupation focused. In the OTIPM, the term *occupation-focused* refers to the degree to which the proximal focus of attention is on occupation.

Traditional task analysis differs from the previous two types of analysis in that it is not occupation focused. Instead, this type of analysis is focused on speculation about the underlying reasons for reduced quality in occupational performance, such as body functions, environmental factors, and other contextual factors. Therefore traditional task analysis is occupation based but not occupation focused.

Finally, *activity analysis* is neither occupation based nor occupation focused. Activity analysis is not occupation based because it is undertaken without observation of the client. When using activity analysis, occupational therapists use the demands of the activity to reason about where the client's performance of the activity is likely to break down. They can then grade and adapt various situational elements such as task elements, temporal elements, and environmental elements accordingly.

In summary, prioritizing true top-down reasoning and observation of the quality of the client's occupational performance is central to *occupational* therapy. The overall goal of the OTIPM is to provide a framework for practice that is occupational and that enables occupational therapists to manifest their distinct area of expertise using occupation-centered reasoning. Fisher and Marterella (2019) asserted that "using the OTIPM inspires occupational therapists to feel renewed pride in their occupational therapy identity, encourages occupational therapists to practice with authenticity, and results in occupational therapists effectively overcoming, or at least minimizing, the various constraints they experience in practice" (p. 4). In the Transactional Model of Occupation, occupation is understood as resulting from a complex situational context in which situational elements combine in a transactional whole that shapes and is shaped by occupation. In the next section, we describe the heart of the OTIPM, the occupational therapy process.

OTIPM: AN INTERVENTION PROCESS MODEL

The OTIPM is an intervention process model that outlines in detail "a practical process for planning and implementing high quality and client-centered occupational therapy services that honor the complexity and power of occupation" (p. 3). While exploring the model, it is important to remember that *the client* could be an individual, a client constellation, a client group, an organization, or a community. As a process model, the OTIPM is organized according to the phases, steps, and actions in the occupational therapy process. There are three phases to the model: evaluation and goal setting, intervention, and reevaluation, which are undertaken in that order. The process is cyclic, and occupational therapists can return to earlier phases as many times as required. Throughout the process, occupational therapists need to develop therapeutic rapport and work collaboratively with the client. They also need to make decisions regarding whether to continue or terminate their services.

The first phase of the OTIPM process is the *evaluation and goal-setting phase*, which has three steps. The first step in this phase is *gather initial information*. Occupational therapists collect information to help them understand the complex relationship between the client's occupations and their situational contexts using the Transactional Model of Occupation. Occupational therapists need to use multiple strategies to elicit this complex information. Examples of information gathering strategies include chart reviews, observation, conversations with clients and others, and occupation-focused interviews. This step encompasses five elements that are addressed in a fluid and often overlapping process and involve understanding (1) what occupations the client identifies as strengths and problems, (2) the situational contexts of the client's occupations, (3) the client's level of participation in society, (4) the client's desired outcomes, and (5) what occupational performances the client wants to prioritize.

The second step in the evaluation and goal-setting phase is *implement performance analyses*. Use of performance analyses is a vital step in a true top-down approach because of the importance of observing and evaluating the quality of a client's occupational performance. There are four sequential components of this step: (1) observe the client's quality of occupational performance, (2) gather the client's perspective on the occupational performance (reported perspective), (3) rate the client's quality of occupational performance (observed perspective), and (4) determine the extent of discrepancy between the observed and reported perspectives on occupational performance. In the OTIPM, a distinction is made between primary and supplementary components of performance analysis. The first and third components are considered primary because these involve observing and rating the quality of the client's occupational performance. The second and fourth components are considered supplementary. They are useful for understanding the client's occupational experiences and being able to make comparisons between the client's perspectives and the occupational therapist's observations, but conducting the supplementary components is not always possible. In a true top-down approach, which emphasizes the actual observation of performance, the client's self-reported experiences do not constitute observation and are therefore considered supplementary. When choosing evaluation methods for this step, Fisher and Marterella (2019) cautioned that, while performance analyses are always occupation based and occupation focused, not all occupation-based and occupation-focused assessments are performance analyses. This is because they do not evaluate performance skills, the smallest observable units of occupation. Fisher and Marterella provided extensive discussion of performance analyses, and readers are encouraged to access *Powerful Practice* for this detailed exploration of evaluation methods.

The third step in the evaluation and goal-setting phase is *finalize evaluation*. This step has three sequential actions: (1) synthesize the findings of the performance analysis, (2) finalize the client's occupation-focused goals, and (3) speculate about the reasons for the client's occupational challenges. First, occupational therapists collate their findings from the previous step and write statements that document the client's baseline level of occupational performance. This includes both challenges and relative strengths; Fisher and Marterella (2019) emphasized that documenting strengths can support an argument for occupational therapy services to build on them. Baseline statements must be observable, and therefore measurable, and should include what was done and how well or effectively it was done. Baseline statements can indicate the client's overall quality of occupational performance, called the *global baseline*, or provide specific baselines based on clusters of performance skills. Quality indicators are used to enable measurement of future performance against baseline performance. These indicators of quality include (1) the type of problem observed, rated according to effort, efficiency, social effectiveness, safety, and independence; and (2) the severity of the problem, rated as no problem, minimal problem, moderate problem, or substantial/marked problem, and according to the temporal aspects of speed or tempo of performance, duration of observed problem, and frequency of observed problem or amount of assistance provided. Baseline statements can also include the client's self-reported performance and the extent of any discrepancy between the quality of observed performance and self-reported performance.

Once the findings of the performance analysis have been synthesized, the second action is to finalize the client's occupation-focused goals. This is done in collaboration with the client and includes clear statements regarding what the client will be able to do and how well they will be able to do it. Fisher and Marterella (2019) discussed the difficulty that can occur in practice when the client is unable to articulate goals or set realistic goals and reminded occupational therapists of their ethical obligation to remain client centered and to promote client engagement in decision-making.

The third action of finalizing evaluation is to speculate about reasons for the client's occupational challenges. For this action, expanded task analysis using the Transactional Model of Occupation is recommended as the most effective option. Using this model helps occupational therapists "to move beyond thinking in terms of underlying body functions, the environment, or other contextual factors as being separate from occupation" (Fisher and Marterella, p. 208) and to base their speculation on a conception of occupation as inextricably intertwined with situational elements in a transactional whole. Thinking this way can be difficult as it differs from the way occupation has traditionally been conceptualized. To aid this change in reasoning and embrace the Transactional Model of Occupation, Fisher and Marterella (2019) provided some reflective questions (pp. 208–210):

- How might the interwoven occupational elements be interacting with and influencing each other and the situational context?
- How might the situational elements be shaping each other and influencing occupation—occupational performance, occupational experience, and participation?
- Have I considered the transactional whole?
- Do I tend to focus on only a few situational elements (e.g., client elements, environmental elements) and ignore others?
- Am I considering the person or occupation as separate from the situational context?
- Am I addressing only occupational performance without considering the interwoven nature of the occupational elements?

The next phase of the OTIPM is the intervention phase. It has one step: *select model(s) of practice, and plan and implement intervention.* In keeping with the overall aim of the OTIPM to promote authentic *occupational* therapy, it identifies four approaches, each with a model of intervention and types of intervention that are legitimate to use. In addition to these four approaches, a fifth, mixed-models approach is added, whereby the intervention approaches can be used in conjunction. When using each intervention approach, collaborative consultation and educational principles are essential features. The first intervention approach includes the *compensatory model* with its associated intervention type, occupation-based and occupation-focused adaptive occupation. This approach is used to compensate for decreased performance skill. Adaptation is a key feature of this approach and can involve introducing temporary or more permanent strategies that are acceptable to the client and to relevant others; can result in task performance that is less effortful, is more efficient, is safe, and reduces the need for assistance; and can increase participation in society. The second approach is based on the *education and teaching model.* This approach involves offering to client groups occupation-focused educational programs such as lectures, workshops, seminars, and in-service programs. These will relate to all aspects of occupation and use occupation-based and/or occupation-focused strategies that consider what people already know and what information would enhance their occupational performance, experience, and participation. The third approach uses the *acquisitional model*. This involves occupation-focused and occupation-based occupational skills training strategies that promote the client's acquisition, redevelopment, and maintenance performance skill. Graded occupation is a core principle in this approach, whereby occupational therapists commence by providing the client with a just-right occupational challenge and then extending that challenge so that the client's skills improve. The fourth approach is guided by the *restorative model*. This approach focuses on "the remediation of underlying impairments, or the restoration, development, or maintenance of underlying body functions or other client elements" (Fisher and Marterella 2019, p. 227). Graded occupation is also a core principle in this approach. Finally, in addition to using one of these for intervention approaches, occupational therapists may choose to use a *mixed-models approach*. They can use more than one model sequentially or simultaneously, depending on occupational therapy goals.

The final phase of the OTIPM is the *reevaluation phase* and the fifth step in the model is *implement reevaluation and ascertain outcomes*. The purpose of this step is to determine whether there has been a change from the recorded baseline statements and whether the client's goals have been met. To determine whether change has occurred, occupational therapists use occupation-based and occupation-focused observations of occupational performance and occupation-focused interviews or self-reports. They compare the quality of previously observed occupational performance with the quality of current occupational performance. In addition, if they had originally gathered information on the supplementary components of performance analysis, they also evaluate whether there has been a change in the discrepancy between observed and reported performance. They also ask the client about their satisfaction with occupation. To determine if the client's level of participation in society has changed they ask questions about the client's engagement in valued occupations, such as (p. 255):

- Are you now more able to engage in activities you feel are necessary or worthwhile?
- Do you feel you are now more able to engage in activities you have committed to or have a responsibility to do?
- When you are engaging in activities in the community, do you feel like you now are able to contribute more, make a bigger difference, or be more helpful to others?
- When you are doing things with others, do you now feel more included, accepted, or socially connected?
- If you have noticed a change in your participation, can you provide more details about that change—has there been a minimal change, a moderate change, or a substantial change?

For the final action in this step, occupational therapists evaluate whether the client's goals have been met and if new goals have been identified. To do this, they make comparisons with the previous baseline statements. The reevaluation phase makes it clear how important it is to document clear and observable baseline statements in the evaluation and goal-setting phase.

In summary, the OTIPM is a process model that uses the Transactional Model of Occupation as its theoretical model. The Transactional Model of Occupation conceptualizes occupation as the *result* of the transaction among seven situational elements. The OTIPM advocates for the use of a true top-down reasoning approach that guides occupational therapists to focus their evaluation on clients' occupational strengths and concerns in their actual contexts and prioritizes occupation and participation in society, thus enabling them to engage in authentic occupational therapy practice. Assessment of the quality of actual occupational performance through performance analyses provides information upon which to speculate how situational and occupational elements are transacting to influence occupational performance, experience, and participation. Box 5.3 continues the case of Alex and Chris, illustrating an OTIPM perspective.

BOX 5.3 ■ OTIPM Case Illustration

After graduating and being employed as an occupational therapist in the same organization where he was a student, Alex was able to continue working with Chris. He started by planning a follow-up meeting to assess Chris's work integration process. They had been employed as a gardener for the last few months, describing that they felt happy and proud of their first job experience. But they also felt frustrated because they were not able to make friends, suspecting that their colleagues were hiding from them. They also reported feeling very tired at the end of the day. Alex decided to assess their work environment and observed Chris for one day in their job. He discovered that Chris works a full day in the main park of the city, where they need to walk long distances. He also observed that, each time Chris works with one of their colleagues on a particular task, Chris gets very anxious. Chris knows they have problems socially and are afraid they might say things that would offend their co-workers.

Looking through the lens of the OTIPM, Alex conducted a performance analysis while observing Chris gardening at their workplace. This showed that, at the activity level, Chris used inappropriate postures to perform gardening tasks, had to walk a long way, was not organized with the tools and materials they needed to use, and was not very efficient in organizing the sequence of the work they needed to complete during the day. Because of the big size of the park the gardeners were located far away from one another, and they did not have a place to share lunch or breaks. What Alex observed was very different from the self-reported assessment Chris completed about their performance. While Chris thought people had been avoiding them, Alex realized the co-workers were simply spread out throughout the park.

Moving forward to the intervention phase, Alex planned to use a compensatory approach to improve Chris's performance and satisfaction with their role as a worker. On Alex's request, the manager agreed to move Chris to a smaller garden where they could receive support from a support worker and could work with some other colleagues who are very sociable. The manager also agreed to grade the integration process, by asking Chris to work only half a day for a while and gradually increasing this until they could work a full day. In relation to the activities that are part of Chris's role, Alex prescribed a small stool so that Chris could sit down while working at ground level and a gardening wagon to carry their tools. When carrying out a reevaluation six months later, Alex found that Chris was completely engaged and satisfied with their role as worker, and their family was proud of them. They told Alex they have been able to buy presents for their sister and parents, which makes them feel worthy and competent.

HISTORICAL DESCRIPTION OF THE MODEL'S DEVELOPMENT

The OTIPM has developed over approximately two decades (Fisher 1998, 2009, 2013; Fisher and Jones 2017; Fisher and Marterella 2019). While the model has been represented by different diagrams at various times, the principles underlying the model have remained consistent and enduring, relating to the question of how to ensure that practice remains truly *occupational*. Fisher explained that the OTIPM grew out of discussions with occupational therapists about everyday practice and her 45 years of experience (Fisher and Jones 2017).

Fisher described studying and practicing occupational therapy during its mechanistic paradigm and being directed to use exercise, neurophysiological approaches, and contrived occupation (e.g., hammering to release emotion) to address underlying impairments (Fisher 1998).

However, during this time, Fisher also experienced firsthand the power of meaningful occupation. She recounted working with a young man who had a spinal cord injury that resulted in quadriplegia. Because he was fascinated by the prospect of building an electronic device, she used a do-it-yourself radio kit as a therapeutic intervention, helping him solve problems related to holding and manipulating objects as he built the radio. In the end, he had a radio to listen to, had satisfaction from his accomplishment, and had learned to develop compensatory strategies to overcome difficulties he encountered. The improvements that occurred in his muscle strength and dexterity were a consequence of engaging in meaningful and purposeful occupation (rather than the focus of the therapy).

Later, Fisher encountered colleagues and mentors who were passionate about using purposeful occupation as a therapeutic medium and centering practice on occupational performance rather than underlying impairments. While she fundamentally believed in this as well, she felt she lacked the vocabulary for explaining the therapeutic value of occupation and the unique contribution of occupational therapy to healthcare. This situation provided the fertile soil for the development of the OTIPM as a framework to guide therapists to be *occupational* in their practice. It was her solution to her long-held puzzle of "how to harness the full power of occupation in practice" (Fisher and Jones 2017, p. 238). She wanted to address three fundamental obstacles to creating a truly occupational practice that she had identified. The first related to the use of decontextualized evaluation methods. About this situation, she asked the following questions: "Why do we evaluate people with sensory integrative dysfunction using decontextualized tests and clinical observations? How do we know that what we are observing is really praxis? How do we know that what we are observing has any relevance to everyday life? Why don't we focus our evaluations on occupational performance?" (Fisher and Jones, p. 238). Second, through observation and discussions with occupational therapists and students, she came to realize that, even when people believed in the power of occupation, they persistently argued for the importance of evaluating and restoring function in underlying impairments as a way of improving clients' abilities to perform tasks in their daily lives. The third obstacle she identified was the difficulty occupational therapists and students expressed regarding how to integrate occupational therapy models and evaluation and intervention methods into practice.

Fisher expressed her passion for the power of occupation. This passion was evident when discussing the notion of occupation. Fisher emphasized that occupation is a "noun of action" (Fisher 1998, p. 511). She described three ways that occupation denotes action. First, "occupation is defined as *the* action of seizing, taking possession of, or occupying space or time"; second, it can signify "*the* holding of an office or position, such as one's role"; and third, it "refers to *the* being engaged in something" (p. 511, italics in original). In relation to enabling clients to engage in the action of seizing, taking possession of, or occupying space and time, occupational therapists need to imagine the spaces such as homes, schools, and workplaces that clients occupy through action in their lives, particularly in relation to the roles they occupy. They need to acknowledge that the performance of tasks involves actions that evolve over time and that occupying time requires engaging in mental, physical, and social tasks that are meaningful to the client. In relation to occupational therapy, she wrote, "[occupation] conveys the powerful essence of our profession — enabling people to perform the actions they need and want to perform so that they can engage in and 'do' the familiar, ordinary, goal-directed activities of every day in a manner that brings meaning and personal satisfaction" (p. 511).

SUMMARY

Powerful Practice aims to assist occupational therapists to maintain authentic, occupational, client-focused practice. Using the Transactional Model of Occupation, occupational therapists view occupation as the *result* of the transaction among situational elements that include the person. It moves away from an individualistic sense of people performing occupation to a nuanced understanding that occupation is always situated in time, place, culture, and relationships, and that the actions of people can only be understood in context. This transactional understanding of occupation is consistent with a general movement in occupational therapy away from a conceptualization of person, occupation, and environment as separate entities and toward a situated whole.

The OTIPM provides a detailed process model that guides occupational therapists through the phases, steps, and actions of an occupational therapy practice based on a transactional appreciation of occupation. Following the process outlined in the OTIPM, occupational therapists can provide services that are characterized by occupation-centered reasoning and top-down thinking and are focused on clients' performance of occupations that are important to them. By centering their practice on occupation, occupational therapists are empowered to contribute their unique perspective and skills.

MEMORY AID

See Box 5.4.

Box 5.4 ■ OTIPM Memory Aid

Is the client an individual, a client constellation, a group, an organization, or a community?
What occupations are meaningful to and priorities for the client? How does the client's participation in society need to be addressed?
Based on observation of their performance and their self-report, what are the client's strengths and problems in relation to their priorities for occupation?
- What occupation-based assessment tools and information gathering methods can help determine this?
For occupations the client has prioritized, how are they influenced by situational elements?
- Temporal—past, present, and future; patterns, sequences, and routines; duration and frequency
- Client—personal factors; embodied habits, routines, rituals, and roles; attitudes, beliefs, interests, and values; occupational priorities; body functions
- Task—expected structure and timing; expected spaces, tools, and materials; intended purpose or outcome
- Physical environment—spaces; tangible objects; digital environments
- Social environment—other people; others' characteristics; others' personal meanings and expectations; pets and service animals; connections and relationships
- Geopolitical—geographical; political; economic; historical
- Sociocultural—rules, regulations, and norms; attitudes and expectations; shared morals, beliefs, values, and customs; ethical considerations
What outcomes will occupational therapy aim to achieve?
What intervention model(s) and associated intervention type(s) will be most appropriate for achieving those outcomes?
- Compensatory model, using occupation-based and occupation-focused adaptive occupation to compensate for decreased occupational performance skill
- Education and teaching model, using occupation-focused educational programs for groups
- Acquisitional model for occupational skills training, using occupation-based and occupation-focused intervention to acquire or redevelop performance skill
- Restorative model for enhancing body functions and other client elements, using occupation-based interventions to restore or develop body functions and other client elements
    Have the outcomes of occupational therapy been achieved? Have new goals been identified?
    Should occupational therapy be continued or terminated?

MAJOR WORKS

Fisher AG, Marterella A. *Powerful Practice: A Model for Authentic Occupational Therapy.* Center for Innovative OT Solutions; 2019.

Conclusion

In this chapter we presented two conceptual frameworks developed in the United States. The Occupational Therapy Practice Framework: Domain and Process (OTPF-4) represents the official position of the American Occupational Therapy Association. The Occupational Therapy Intervention Process Model (OTIPM) was developed by Anne Fisher over several decades. Both center on occupation as the core concern of occupational therapy theory and practice. They emphasize the importance of identifying the occupations that are meaningful to clients in the context of their daily lives and of working collaboratively with them. They also conceptualize occupation as richly contextualized, with the OTIPM using the Transactional Model of Occupation as a conceptual model explaining that occupation is the result of the transaction among seven situational elements. The OTPF highlights occupational justice as an issue central to a contextualized understanding of occupation.

As a practice framework and a process model, respectively, the OTPF and the OTIPM attend to the process used by occupational therapists, guiding them step by step through this process. Each outlines a process for information gathering that involves attention to occupational performance and participation in daily life in society, with the OTIPM emphasizing the need for observation of the client's actual performance. They both include the step of synthesizing the data collected. Through this process, occupational therapists ensure that they have a comprehensive understanding of the client's occupational needs before collaboratively setting goals for occupational therapy service. They both outline common approaches to intervention: in the OTPF the approaches are to create or promote, establish or restore, maintain, modify, and prevent; in the OTIPM the approaches use the compensatory model, education and teaching model, acquisitional model, and restorative model. Both end the process with determination of whether the established outcomes have been achieved and whether occupational therapy services should be terminated or continued.

References

AOTA. Occupational therapy product output reporting system and uniform terminology for reporting occupational therapy services, 1979. Available from pracdept@aota.org.

AOTA. Uniform terminology for occupational therapy—second edition. *Am J Occup Ther.* 1989 Dec;43(12):808–815. doi:10.5014/ajot.43.12.808

AOTA. Uniform terminology for occupational therapy—third edition. American Occupational Therapy Association. *Am J Occup Ther.* 1994 Nov-Dec;48(11):1047–1054. doi:10.5014/ajot.48.11.1047

AOTA. Occupational therapy practice framework: domain and process. *Am J Occup Ther.* 2002 Nov-Dec;56(6):609–639.

AOTA. Occupational therapy practice framework: domain and process-second edition. *Am J Occup Ther.* 2008 Nov-Dec;62:625–683.

AOTA. Occupational therapy practice framework: domain and process-third edition. *Am J Occup Ther.* 2014 Mar-Apr;68(Suppl. 1):625–683.

AOTA. Occupational therapy practice framework: domain and process—fourth edition. *Am J Occup Ther.* 2020 Aug 1;74(Supplement_2):7412410010p1–7412410010p87. doi:10.5014/ajot.2020.74S2001

Dickie V, Cutchin MP, Humphry R. Occupation as transactional experience: a critique of individualism in occupational science. *J Occup Science.* 2006 Apr;13(1):83–93. doi:10.1080/14427591.2006.9686573

Fisher AG. Uniting practice and theory in an occupational framework – 1998. Eleanor Clarke Slagle Lecture. *Am J Occup Ther.* 1998;52:509–521. doi:10.5014.aot.52.7.509

Fisher AG. *Occupational Therapy Intervention Process Model: A Model for Planning and Implementing Top-Down, Client-Centered, and Occupation-Based Interventions.* Three Star Press; 2009.

Fisher AG. Occupation-centred, occupation-based, occupation-focused: same, same, or different? *Scand J Occup Ther.* 2013 May;20(3):162–173. doi:10.3109/11038128.2012.754492

Fisher AG, Jones KB. Occupational Therapy Intervention Process Model. In: Hinojosa J, Kramer P, Royeen CB, eds. *Perspectives on Human Occupation: Theories Underlying Practice*. 2nd ed. Wolters Kluwer/ Lippincott Williams & Wilkins; 2017:237–286.

Fisher AG, Marterella A. *Powerful Practice: A Model for Authentic Occupational Therapy*. Center for Innovative OT Solutions; 2019.

Nilsson I, Townsend E. Occupational justice—bridging theory and practice. *Scand J Occup Ther*. 2010;17(1):57–63. doi:10.3109/11038120903287182

World Federation of Occupational Therapists (WFOT). 2023. About occupational therapy. Retrieved 5/04/2023 from https://www.wfot.org/about/about-occupational-therapy.

CHAPTER 6

The Model of Human Occupation (MOHO)

CHAPTER CONTENTS

Main Concepts and Definitions of
Terms   113
　Volition   114
　Habituation   117
　Performance Capacity and the Lived
　Body   120
　Environment   122
Dimensions of Doing   124
A Narrative Approach to the Lifespan   125

Pathways of Change in MOHO   126
Use of the Model in Practice   127
Historical Description of the Model's
Development   130
Memory Aid   133
Conclusion   134
References   135

The Model of Human Occupation (Kielhofner 1985, 1995, 2002, 2008; Taylor 2017), or MOHO as it is known, is the longest published model in occupational therapy. MOHO has been very influential over its long history. According to Taylor (2017), it is "the most widely used occupation-focused model in occupational therapy practice in the United States and internationally" (p. 5). At the time it was first published, the major occupational therapy models available in North America were occupational performance models (see Chapter 3). MOHO provided a unique perspective that differed from those models. Whereas occupational performance models primarily focused on physical rehabilitation, MOHO addressed issues relevant to other areas of practice, such as those dealing with conditions that were permanent and required a focus broader than rehabilitation. MOHO provided an approach to the concept of human occupation that was quite broad, focusing on "a client's engagement and participation in occupations as a mechanism of change" (p. 5). It provided a unique perspective, introducing novel concepts such as *volition* and *habituation* to occupational therapy models, concepts that have been incorporated into more recent versions of models and frameworks.

Main Concepts and Definitions of Terms

In this chapter we present the fifth edition of MOHO (Taylor 2017), which is the first edition of the text not edited by Gary Kielhofner. However, many of the chapters include Kielhofner as a posthumous author. The model has evolved and changed substantially over its five editions, reflecting both a development in its understanding of human occupation and the context of an ever-changing world in which different perspectives and values have been prominent at different times. Some of the changes to MOHO over time are captured in the section "Historical Description of the Model's Development," later in this chapter.

MOHO provides a theoretical framework for understanding the concept of human occupation. Human occupation is defined as "the doing of work, play, or activities of daily living within a temporal, physical, and sociocultural context that characterizes much of human life" (Taylor 2017, p. 9). It refers to the everyday things people do that give them meaning and identity. While concerned with the broad concept of human occupation, MOHO also makes a temporal distinction between activities and occupation. While activities are the things people move in and out of each day and throughout the day, occupation refers to larger patterns of activity such as roles, habit patterns, and personal projects (all of which contribute to the attribution of meaning and development of identity). MOHO provides a theoretical framework that explains how occupation is selected, organized, and undertaken within the actual contexts in which people live.

While MOHO distinguishes between person and environment, it takes a transactional approach based on dynamic systems theory. The diagram used in the fifth edition presents MOHO as a nucleus surrounded by the four elements of volition, habituation, performance capacity, and environment. These four elements interact in an equal and mutually influencing way to determine the nature of a person's occupational engagement, thus creating a whole, dynamic system. This person-in-environment system has the capacity to self-organize when needed. According to O'Brien and Kielhofner (2017), this dynamic system moves through "fluctuations of continuity and change, particularly non-linear forms of change" (p. 25). Reference to changes that are nonlinear highlights that, in dynamic systems theory, a change in one or more elements of the system prompts a change in the whole system that cannot be predicted (as distinct from a linear cause–effect relationship in which the effect can be anticipated from the cause). While people generally prefer continuity to change, when the person-in-environment system becomes sufficiently destabilized a change is required. O'Brien and Kielhofner referred to such a disturbance as a *perturbation*. They explained that perturbations can be external to the person (e.g., the loss of a job) or internal (e.g., a sense of discomfort). Because dynamic systems have the capacity to self-organize, perturbations will prompt new interactions and relationships between various components of the system, creating a new and transformed equilibrium (i.e., the system reaches a new steady state that is different from its previous steady state). When applied to the dynamic person-in-environment system, occupation is facilitated when all four elements are working well together. While minor disturbances in the person-in-environment interaction might not be experienced as problems, or even noticed, major perturbations will be experienced as occupational problems. Solving these occupational problems requires the establishment of a new steady state, in which the four elements of the person-in-environment system reconfigure their interaction to establish a new equilibrium.

As we turn now to a more detailed discussion of the four elements of MOHO, it is important to keep dynamic systems theory in mind. While we consider each element separately, it is important to remember that they are inextricably and mutually connected, forming a whole that is more than the sum of its parts. For example, Yamada et al. (2017) stated, "within MOHO, consideration of any aspect of the person (volition, habituation, and performance) always includes how the environment is influencing the person's motivation, pattern, and performance. The environment is a constant influence on occupation, and persons' occupational circumstances cannot be appreciated without an understanding of their environments" (p. 11). To aid readers to navigate the following sections, Table 6.1 provides a list of the four elements and their components.

VOLITION

Volition refers to the motivation that underpins occupation. People are assumed to have a need or desire to act in the world as well as distinct thoughts and feelings about what they do. In MOHO,

TABLE 6.1 ■ **Elements and Components**

Volition
- Volitional process—anticipate, choose, experience, interpret (through reflection)
- Personal causation—sense of personal capacity, self-efficacy
- Values—personal convictions, sense of obligation
- Interests

Habituation
- Habits—habits of occupational performance, habits of routine, habits of style
- Internalized roles

Performance Capacity and the Lived Body
- Performance capacity—objective and subjective components
- The lived body—mind-body unity

Environment
- Physical environment—space, objects
- Social environment—relationships, interactions
- Occupational environment—occupations, activities

volition is conceptualized as having three interconnected components as well as a volitional process. The three well-known components of volition in MOHO are *personal causation*, defined as "one's sense of capacity and effectiveness"; *values*, which refers to what people find "important and meaningful to do"; and *interests*, indicating what people find "enjoyable and satisfying to do" (Yamada et al. 2017, p. 12). These relate to what a person feels they can do, what has relevance to them, and what interests them in the context of their situation, and all influence their motivation for occupation. We first discuss the volitional process and then these components of volition.

The *volitional process* refers to the sequence whereby people experience, interpret, anticipate, and choose occupations. The process introduces the temporal aspects of volition, in that people first experience something and then interpret it as they reflect on it. Then they anticipate what they might do when they are presented with the possibility of acting immediately and in the distant future, and they make activity and occupational choices. Finally, they choose what activities they will enter and exit at the time or in the immediate future. They also make occupational choices when they make longer-term commitments. As Yamada et al. explained, "Ordinarily, occupational choices require some deliberation and may involve information gathering, reflection, imagining possibilities, and considering alternatives" (p. 14). Over time, as people have new experiences and reflect on them, changes occur in the ways they think about themselves and their lives. These then lead to changes in what they anticipate and choose to do. A cycle then develops as these choices regarding activities and occupation lead to new experiences and reflections, and so on. Changes can be small or large and can serve to reinforce or alter people's sense of agency, values, and interests. These cycles of change continue throughout people's lives. Even when people appear to have substantial stability in their lives, there are always at least incremental changes that occur through this repeated volitional process. Lee and Kielhofner (2017a) summarized the reciprocal nature of the process by explaining that, when this process is repeated, it maintains or reshapes a person's personal causation, values, and interests.

We now turn to the components of volition: personal causation, values, and interests. While each of these components is detailed separately, Lee and Kielhofner (2017a) emphasized that they must be understood as aspects of a larger volitional whole in which they are dynamically interconnected and mutually influencing. Depending upon people's circumstances and perspectives, some volitional components may be more influential than others.

The first volitional component, *personal causation*, refers to a person's sense of both what they are capable of doing and the effectiveness of their actions. These two dimensions, respectively, are referred to and defined in MOHO as "the sense of personal capacity [which] is a self-assessment of one's physical, intellectual, and social abilities" and "self-efficacy, [which] refers to one's sense of effectiveness in using personal capacities to achieve desired outcomes in life" (Lee and Kielhofner 2017a, p.42). When people feel both capable and effective, they are motivated to act. But, depending on people's circumstances and history, either or both can be limited, which can affect their motivation for action. People's sense of personal capacity and self-efficacy develops over the course of their lives, with their various experiences enhancing or diminishing these dimensions. They are specific to various aspects of people's lives, in that people can feel they have a certain agency (capacity and effectiveness) in some circumstances and not others. The two also develop in the context of a culture that determines what actions are acceptable, when, and by whom.

The overall concept of personal causation relates to an individual's perceptions of their own ability to achieve their goals and to affect their own lives and those of others. People's motivation for action depends on what they believe they can achieve. They are more likely to do what they think is possible for them and important to do. However, people's beliefs can differ from objective evaluations of their capacities. People can overestimate or underestimate their capacities to act and effect change within their actual context. Overestimation can lead to injury and other negative consequences and underestimation may lead to people unnecessarily limiting their actions. When there are changes in people's capacities—for example, through illness or injury—it may take time for them to discover what they can do and to form realistic beliefs about their own changed capacities. If they have a progressive condition, planning for the future can be difficult because of an unknown sense of what their own capacities will be.

The second volitional component is *values*. In MOHO, the concept of values refers to the beliefs and convictions people have about "what is good, right, and important to do" (Lee and Kielhofner 2017a, p.46). Values develop within cultural contexts that convey messages about how people should act and what they should strive for. These cultural contexts include broader levels such as society and narrower systems such as social groups and families, and values can be passed on from generation to generation. Values become internalized by people, often without conscious awareness. These internalized values, in turn, determine the sense of self-worth a person derives from what they do. Lee and Kielhofner explained that, when people perform in culturally meaningful and sanctioned ways, they feel valued as members of the cultural group. When not conforming to cultural expectations, they can feel "shame, guilt, failure, or inadequacy" (p. 46).

MOHO identifies both *personal convictions* and a *sense of obligation* as contributing to people's values and their consequent actions. Personal convictions derive from people's world views and are defined as "strongly held views of life that define what matters" (Lee and Kielhofner 2017a, p.46). People's convictions reside deep within them, and they generally act according to those convictions. In contrast, when they feel they are acting contrary to those convictions, they often feel deep shame. People's beliefs about how they *should* act relate to their sense of obligation. People often feel obligations to others and to organizations and social institutions. As with personal convictions, failure to fulfill their obligations can cause people to negatively evaluate themselves.

The third volitional component is *interest*. Interests are defined as "what one finds enjoyable or satisfying to do" (Lee and Kielhofner 2017a, p. 48). Interests are abundantly diverse and individual, flowing from people's experiences and their reflections upon those experiences. If certain experiences result in enjoyment, people are likely to seek similar experiences again. However, they are likely to avoid experiences they did not find enjoyable in the past. Over time, patterns of interests develop. These patterns contribute to the anticipation and choosing of activities that align with interests. Depending upon their circumstances, some people may have more opportunity than others to engage in activities they find enjoyable and satisfying. In general, engagement in enjoyable and satisfying activities has a positive effect on health. However, Lee and Kielhofner noted that some activities that give pleasure can also become problematic for people. They gave examples of people engaging in socially unacceptable activities or interests that are harmful, such as overuse of alcohol and substance abuse.

Lee and Kielhofner (2017a) discussed how the three volitional components—personal causation, values, and interests—contribute to the volitional process, which involves anticipation, making choices, having experiences, and evaluating and interpreting them by reflecting on them. Regarding anticipation, personal causation, values, and interests determine what people seek and notice. If something is not important to them, they tend not to notice it. If people feel they can make a difference to something that is important to them and aligns with their interests, they are more likely to determine opportunities for acting meaningfully. It is by anticipating their own agency, commitments, and interests that they make choices about what to do in the short and long terms. In the short term, they make decisions about what activities to do and how to do them. They also make longer-term choices about occupation (e.g., changes to roles and habits). Occupational choices occur less frequently than activity choices, which are made constantly throughout the day, and require people's considered deliberation because of the substantial impact these decisions can have on their lives. Once people have made choices regarding which activities and occupations to engage in, they experience and interpret them. Their personal causation, values, and interests will shape their experiences and interpretations. For example, their experiences will be influenced by how much impact they feel they can make, how important these activities and occupations are to achieving their purposes, and how much enjoyment and satisfaction they derive from them. If they experience activities and occupations positively, they are more likely to interpret them as worth repeating in the future. If any of the components of volition are less positively evaluated, the activity or occupation is most likely to be interpreted as requiring a change. Lee and Kielhofner emphasized that life satisfaction is enhanced when there is harmony between what people do in their lives and their volitional thoughts and feelings.

HABITUATION

The second element of MOHO is *habituation*. Habituation is defined as "an internalized readiness to exhibit consistent patterns of behavior guided by our habits and roles and fitted to the characteristics of routine temporal, physical, and social environments" (Lee and Kielhofner 2017b, p. 57). At the core of this definition is an intimate relationship between people and their environments. Lee and Kielhofner (2017b) referred to this as "interdependency of habituation and habitat" (p. 59). Regarding people, they need to be "ready" to develop behavioral routines and to sense opportunities for these. Rather than approaching every activity anew, people develop patterns of behavior that reduce their cognitive load when engaged in activities. Regarding environments, activities are conducted in specific contexts and the development of behavioral patterns requires adequate alignment with these contexts. Achieving alignment depends on the stability of those environments. If environments are constantly changing, so too are the demands of the activities undertaken within them, thus preventing these activities from becoming routinized and habitual. Instead, they will constantly require conscious attention. In contrast, stable environments provide a level of predictability, enabling activities to be undertaken with less conscious effort when they are repeated and behavioral routines to develop.

Habituation has two components: habits and internalized roles. *Habits* are defined as "acquired tendencies to automatically respond and perform in certain, consistent ways in familiar environments or situations" (Lee and Kielhofner 2017b, p. 60). Habits are about doing things automatically and consistently. As explained, to be able to act automatically, environments need a familiarity. When environments are familiar, people can generally respond with habitual action.

This action is patterned and embodied and requires little conscious attention. However, when environments are less familiar, greater conscious attention is required for engaging in activities in that context. People are unable to act in habitual ways because they need to continually plan and assemble action in new ways to accommodate for the differing demands of the environment.

Habits also develop over time, building on previous performance. Some habits develop from childhood as children learn routines and incorporate social mores and expectations. Some habits remain relatively stable throughout life while others change as people develop and take on new roles. However, habits are generally resistant to change because they are based on an individual's fundamental worldview and expectations (which are generally quite stable) about how the world is ordered. Therefore, when new habits are required for responding to new environments, they are often based on old and established habits, which are modified to suit the new environment. Habitual ways of doing things are generally efficient because they require minimal conscious effort (allowing attention to be directed elsewhere) and encompass skills that have developed through practice and become embodied. Because they use bodily memory and free up conscious attention, they enable engagement in more than one thing at a time (e.g., dressing while planning for the day, walking while talking on the telephone). As Lee and Kielhofner summed up, "habits hold together the patterns of ordinary action that give life its familiar and relatively effortless character" (p. 60).

Habits are not just individual. When they are shared by a group of people, they form the basis of social customs. When internalized by people as habits, social customs allow for the smooth functioning of society and individuals act in predictable and socially meaningful ways. These social customs can be acquired by individuals and passed to others in the social group, whereby the habits of one individual can provide the environment for the habitual behaviors of others. Lee and Kielhofner (2017b) gave the example of one elderly man developing the habit of collecting his mail at a regular time in the morning. As other elderly men commenced the same habit, a regular informal gathering of elderly men developed in which they would talk and spend the morning together. This anecdote illustrates the close and mutually influencing association between social customs and individual habits and that people's actions are embedded within specific environments and social contexts. People and environments are inextricably linked, shaping and being shaped by one another. People's habitual ways of doing things influence the context as their social and physical environments respond to their actions. Conversely, these environments place demands on individuals to respond from their repertoire of habits or develop new habits. Culture pervades this two-way influencing.

Lee and Kielhofner (2017b) identified three types of habits. *Habits of occupational performance* relate to how people perform routine activities. As people repeat activities, they generally undertake them in a consistent way, with refinement through practice. Over time, as activities are repeated and refined, performance becomes habitual and embodied and requires little or no conscious attention. Most people can identify activities that they undertake without thinking. Some activities are performed so automatically that people might not even remember having done them. A common example involves people being unable to remember if they had locked the door when leaving the house and, when going back to check, finding that they had locked it without being aware of what they were doing. *Habits of routine* introduce the temporal dimension of habits. Routines give shape to people's lives. For example, routines might relate to the time of day (e.g., morning routines), the time of the week (e.g., the working week and weekends in industrialized societies), the time of year (e.g., seasons, school terms), and so forth. Temporally organized routines often relate to social roles—for example, preparing for and ending a period of work (role of worker), getting children off to school in time (role of parent), and attending a scheduled medical appointment (role of client). *Habits of style* indicate that people have their own unique ways of being in the world, their own dispositions and personalities. Each person has a different character which determines how they act. For example, one person might be impatient and do things quickly and immediately, and another might be meticulous and careful or hesitant and cautious.

The second component of habituation is *internalized roles*. This component particularly emphasizes that human occupation is embedded in context. Participation in society is generally organized according to social roles and their associated role status and expectations about relationships and what to do. People internalize these role expectations, which, in turn, affect their identity and beliefs about the actions appropriate to the role. They think of themselves as, for example, a spouse, a friend, a student, or a worker and they associate specific activities and responsibilities with those roles. In addition, the feedback they gain from others regarding their performance of a role shapes their identity.

Lee and Kielhofner (2017b) defined internalized roles as "the incorporation of a socially and/ or personally defined status and a character cluster of attitudes and actions" (p. 65). This definition emphasizes that roles are determined by the interaction between social and personal expectations. In any society, shared meanings and sociocultural expectations develop regarding specific roles. Some roles are more highly valued than others, and roles vary with expectations such as the level of skill or responsibility required. Individuals also have varying expectations about what a particular role requires of them. They will have different motivations regarding the role, and these will shape how they go about conducting it. For example, one person might try to conduct the role well to achieve recognition and gain a sense of pride. Another person might approach the same role with expediency and fulfill it as quickly as possible. When a specific person adopts a particular role, internal and external conceptualizations of the role combine. The result is that any two people will define and approach a certain role differently, and the expectations of any role will vary according to specific societies, social groups, and institutions.

People learn the role expectations of societies and groups through the process of socialization. This process can occur in childhood or when people are new to a sociocultural context. People learn what is expected and proscribed, often by observing and obtaining feedback on their own behavior. Over the course of people's lives, role socialization generally moves from informal to formal. For example, young children are generally socialized and undertake their roles in a wide variety of informal ways. As they grow, their socialization becomes more formal, typically being supported by teachers and supervisors and involving education and training programs that lead to formal qualifications.

Social roles provide the primary vehicle for organizing what people do. Therefore, because a person's configurations of roles vary at different times of their lives, the activities in which they engage will also change. For example, the activities required of a student differ from those of a worker and the activities people will engage in will be determined by their multiple concurrent roles. Changes in roles also prompt alterations in behavior. For example, people change the way they dress, speak, and relate to others when they relinquish roles or adopt new ones. Role change also alters the way people use their time. For example, one role might require that certain activities are done at a particular time, and multiple roles that are undertaken simultaneously will require people to engage in several activities at the same time. Roles also change over the life course, with some roles being associated with certain stages of life. For example, in Western societies people are generally expected to move through the sequence of primary life roles of young child, school and postschool student, worker, and retiree. Other common life roles such as spouse and parent are associated with early and middle adulthood. Throughout their lives, people also move in and out of other short-term and informal roles. When people change their roles during the course of their lives, the process is referred to as *role transition*. Normative role transitions occur at times during the life course that are expected and socially sanctioned. Some role transitions are non-normative, in that they are out of step with social expectations. These are often not chosen and can be distressing and have far-reaching negative consequences.

Lee and Kielhofner (2017b) emphasized that roles are central to the development of self-identity. People's perceptions of themselves generally develop through their experiences of role performance. They form a sense of their own skills and abilities, their personality and dispositions, their preferences and likes and dislikes. Some roles are more self-defining than others. People are likely to seek out roles that align well with their sense of personal causation, values, and interests. However, other roles "just need to be done" and contribute little to the person's sense of identity (except, for example, for people who identify as "a person who gets things done"). When a role affords valued social status and social positioning, it is often tied closely to personal identity. Consequently, a person might go to extraordinary lengths to keep such a role, hence maintaining their social status and preserving their personal identity. Other roles are informally held and generally do not attract a high social status. Because they are less tightly defined by society, people have greater opportunity and responsibility to define and mold them (i.e., make the roles their own). Because obtaining social feedback is important for personal identity development, people who are informally holding roles often need to recruit social partners to validate the role and determine reasonable expectations. Overall, people engage in a variety of roles, both formally and informally. While some roles might contribute more to a person's self-identity than others, it is the combination of roles that contributes to a person's overall sense of identity.

When roles are disrupted or lost, or people are prevented from accessing social roles because of social discrimination, identity and self-esteem can be substantially reduced. As Lee and Kielhofner (2017b) stated, "without sufficient roles one lacks identity, purpose, and structure in everyday life" (p. 68). They explained that psychosocial well-being is adversely affected by limited access to roles with, for example, unemployment being associated with mental and stress-related physical health problems. They summarized the issue by saying, "there is a substantial cost to personal identity when persons no longer are recognized as the fathers, mothers, spouses, students, workers, caretakers, or friends that they used to be" (p. 68). Some people, because of social categorizations such as disabled or the many other varieties of difference, are prevented from engaging in valued social roles. They are relegated to devalued roles such as sick, deviant, and disabled. Frequent social assumptions about people with visible signs of disability are that they are incapable and in need of protection and help. When these negative assumptions become internalized, a person's self-identity can incorporate such assumptions of helplessness and dependence (because feedback is important to identity development). Lee and Kielhofner illustrated this internalization by presenting an excerpt from Zola's (1982) personal account of using a wheelchair. After recounting being treated as incapable by others, he stated, "most frightening was my own compliance, my alienation from myself and from the process" (p. 52). He then described how he avoided contact with other people with a chronic disease or physical disability to enable him to construct an identity through other associations.

PERFORMANCE CAPACITY AND THE LIVED BODY

In this third component of MOHO, the focus moves from the volition for action and the habits and roles that organize action to the action itself. In MOHO, action is discussed in terms of the capacity for performance and the embodied experience of performance.

People's ability to engage in occupation depends upon a match between the demands of the environment and the capacities of the person. A person's *performance capacity* is defined as "the ability to do things provided by the status of underlying objective physical and mental components and corresponding subjective experience" (Tham et al. 2017, p. 75). MOHO conceptualizes performance capacity as having *objective and subjective components*. The objective components of performance capacity can be measured and observed. These include the capacities of body systems such as musculoskeletal, neurological, and cardiopulmonary, as well as cognitive and perceptual processes and so forth. Unlike the earlier occupational performance models, MOHO does not provide details of the elements of performance capacity, recommending instead that other frameworks be used to inform exploration of performance capacity. Examples of these include biomechanical, motor control, sensory, and cognitive frameworks. These frameworks provide guidance for systematically observing and measuring a person's capacities. Knowledge of any structural and functional problems can be used to anticipate difficulties people are likely to have in performing everyday activities and to inform rehabilitation. Tham et al. presented the objective perspective gained from assessment and observation of objective components of performance as the "view from outside" (p. 77). In contrast to this outside view, people experience their own capacities in unique ways. Tham et al. referred to the subjective perspective of performance as the "view from inside" (p. 77). Listening to and trying to understand the subjective experience of a person's own capacities is important for gaining a richer understanding of performance capacity overall. While both perspectives contribute to a holistic understanding of performance, Tham et al. commented that, even when therapists explore their clients' subjective appearances, their goal is usually to build their objective understanding more fully. This hints at the long period of objectification of the body that has been prevalent in health services in the post–World War II period. While subjective experience has been acknowledged throughout the move from a biomedical model to a biopsychosocial model, an emphasis on the objective identification of bodily impairments runs deep.

Tham et al. (2017) explained that this highly valued focus on the body is a consequence of the mind-body dualism, prevalent in Western societies since the time of the philosopher Descartes early in the Enlightenment period. The mind-body dualism posits that the mind and body are distinct and different entities. The body is understood as a physical object with observable properties, such as size, weight, and ability to move through space, that should be studied using the methods of the physical sciences. In contrast, the mind consists of mental properties such as consciousness (e.g., the ability to think and feel) and intentionality (e.g., values and beliefs). While bodily properties are externally observable, mental properties are internal and subjective. Tham et al. advocated for adopting the alternative perspective of *mind-body unity,* in which the mind and body are perceived as an integrated whole. However, they explained that this conceptual shift is difficult because "dualism is deeply ingrained in our way of thinking" (p. 78). They proposed that considering both how the body is experienced and how the mind is embodied are useful strategies for facilitating this integrated understanding.

When considering how the body is experienced, MOHO uses the concept of *the lived body*, a term borrowed from phenomenology (a discipline of philosophy), to refer to embodied experience (i.e., the body as lived). This concept has been used in occupational therapy to refer to the embodied experience of performance, whereby people live and move in a specific body that shapes their experience of performance.

People experience their bodies in two ways: as object and as subject. The less common way that bodies and body parts can be experienced is as objects. People can be conscious of and observe their bodies as they move. For example, people can be aware of turning their head or watching their arm as it reaches out in front of them. However, the second, more common, way that the body is experienced is through its interaction with the world. Rather than a person's attention being directed toward the body, it is directed toward a desired goal. This might be to pick up a glass, clean a mirror, drive a car, or walk to the shop to buy milk. While the body is engaged in all these activities, and becomes the avenue through which they are enacted, the movements themselves are not the focus of attention. People experience the activity involved in pursuing the goal, and the body's contribution remains largely unnoticed. The body forms the invisible background against which people attend to the activities they are performing. As Tham et al. (2017) summarized, "the fundamental difference between experiencing our bodies as object and as subject goes as follows: when I experience some part of my body as an object in the world, I am attending to that body part and am distinguishing between my body and myself. When I am attending to the world from my body, there is no distinction between self and body" (p. 78). The authors then referred to Jean-Paul Sartre's assertion that a person does not just *have* a body but *is* their body. A person's experience is embodied.

From this perspective, the body is largely the taken-for-granted means through which people engage with and experience the world. In phenomenology, this everyday experience is called *the natural attitude*. The body becomes the standpoint *through* which the world is experienced. Experience is inherently embodied. It is only when the body cannot carry out activity effortlessly that it becomes the focus of attention and becomes objectified (e.g., when disabled or injured, or the demands of the task exceed the body's capacities).

To understand how the mind is embodied, because the mind is associated with knowing in dualistic thinking, the phenomenon of knowing provides an excellent focus. Tham et al. (2017) discussed two ways of knowing: knowing things and knowing how to do things. Both are essentially embodied processes. Everything that people know and learn about is created through an interaction between their body and the world. People know about the world through their senses. Even when learning facts, they encounter the information by reading a book or listening to someone or something. During this process of acquiring knowledge, the body remains unnoticed, and attention is focused outwardly on the activity. People are not aware of the process the body has played in the process of acquiring knowledge. The same occurs with knowing how to do things. Learning how to do something involves acquiring knowledge and developing skill through reading, listening, and repeated practice and refinement. While attention can be directed toward a part of the body while aiming to refine a skill, knowing how to do something becomes an embodied form of knowing. This becomes especially obvious when people are asked to describe how to do something. It is often very difficult to describe in words how to do things, and people frequently find themselves acting it out and then reporting what they are doing. Similarly, when teaching others, it can be very frustrating to correct them through language alone and, often, showing them or using hand-on-hand strategies is easier. In both ways of knowing, the body is always the vehicle through which people come to know. Knowledge is always embodied.

A lived body perspective on performance (based on mind-body unity) emphasizes people's experience of engaging in activities. Rather than being aware of the movements they are performing, embodied experience places them *within* those movements. Performance is often disrupted when too much conscious attention is directed to the movements involved. Generally, when learning something new, greater conscious attention is required, but once it becomes an embodied skill, it can be performed automatically without conscious attention and becomes habitual.

ENVIRONMENT

The fourth element of the person-in-environment dynamic system of MOHO is the *environment*. Before turning to a discussion of the environment, Fisher et al. (2017) provided a reminder that, when dynamic systems are working well, the elements align and interact well to achieve the system's purposes. All elements are mutually influencing, and the system can reorganize itself as required to achieve its purposes. When applied to human occupation, if volition, habituation, performance capacity, and the demands of the environment do not align to facilitate occupation, any or all of these elements and their unique configuration can be changed to enable occupation. The changes required might be small or large, and changes in one element will also create changes in the others. The environments in which people conduct their everyday lives can promote or hinder occupation and participation. Environments can impede participation for specific individuals when there is a poor fit with their motivations and abilities, and for groups of people and categories of people (e.g., disabled people; people of a specific age, gender, or ethnicity) when there are structural aspects of the environment that are exclusionary.

MOHO defines the environment as "the particular physical, social, occupational, economic, political, and cultural components of one's contexts that impact upon the motivation, organization, and performance of occupation" (Fisher et al. 2017, p. 93). The model identifies three dimensions of the environment: physical, social, and occupational. It also emphasizes that, simultaneously, people's lives are influenced by their economic, political, cultural, social, geographical, and ecological contexts.

Fisher et al. (2017) provided a detailed table of examples of each of the three environmental dimensions, outlining their components and qualities (we only provide a few examples here, see Fisher et al. 2017, pp. 94–95, for a more detailed list). The first dimension, the *physical environment*, comprises the components of space and objects. Examples of space include streetscapes, buildings and their interiors, and outdoor spaces such as gardens, parks, paths, and various aspects of the countryside. Examples of objects include tools and equipment, clothing and possessions, assistive technology, and vehicles and public transportation. Qualities of the physical environment include accessibility, safety, adequacy, and choice of space; visual and cognitive supports; sensory qualities; overall appearance; and availability and adequacy of objects. The second dimension, the *social environment*, encompasses the components of relationships and interactions. Examples of the different groups of people with whom a person might have relationships include family, social networks, and community members. Examples of types of interactions include verbal communication, nonverbal communication, and pictures, as well as physical and cognitive support and facilitation. The qualities of the social environment include availability of people and relationships, emotional support, empowerment, physical and cognitive facilitation, form of interaction, adequacy of communication, and community and broader social attitudes and services (see Fisher et al. 2017, p. 95, for detailed examples). The components of the third environmental dimension, the *occupational environment*, include occupations, activities, and their properties. Occupations and activities include the usual occupational therapy categories as well as using electronic devices and participating in community organizations, healthcare, and rehabilitation. Qualities of the occupational environment include occupation and activity choices, appeal of occupations and activities, supports available, qualities of participation, time elements, structure, flexibility, sustainability, cultural aspects, and funding and policies (see Fisher et al. 2017, p. 95, for detailed examples).

The various environments within which people's everyday lives are embedded shape how they live. These environments are complex and constantly changing. From moment to moment, environments can afford and constrain occupational participation and influence how activities are undertaken by placing demands on performance in that environment. The person-in-environment is a dynamic system in which all components must work together to achieve a desired outcome regarding occupational performance and participation. When environments and people's volition and performance capacities are stable, people are often able to repeat activities and develop habits and routines. However, if even one aspect of this dynamic person-in-environment system alters, people need to find new ways of performing their activities. For example, people commonly have routines for undertaking self-care activities in their own homes. However, when in a different environment, perhaps at a friend's house or on holidays, the altered demands of a new environment will require them to undertake those same activities in a different way. When changes occur in aspects of a person—perhaps their motivations and goals or their capacities for performance have changed—other aspects of the person-in-environment system will need to alter in accordance. This will most likely require either adjustments to the way activities are performed or modifications to how the environment is organized, or both.

Fisher et al. (2017) used the term *environmental impact* to refer to "the opportunity, support, demand, and constraint that the environment has on a particular individual" and they explained that whether these "are noticed or felt depends on each person's current values, interests, personal causation, roles, habits, and performance capacities" (p. 98). When providing examples of environmental impact, they referred to the work on flow theory of Csikszentmihalyi (Nakamura and Csikszentmihalyi 2014). This theory links the experience of performance to the degree of alignment between a person's capacities and the demands of the environment. In this theory, people become completely absorbed (or experience flow) and are largely unaware of time passing when environmental demands provide an optimal challenge. If a person's capacities far exceed the demands of the environment, the person will feel bored and disengaged, and time will seem to pass slowly. If environmental demands are too high, the person will feel stressed and overwhelmed, and might feel that there is insufficient time. Environments also impose barriers that limit occupational participation in society and the authors referred to the social model of disability to illustrate this. In that model, disability results from environments that present barriers and are therefore disabling. The barriers imposed could relate to the physical environment—for example, stairs, broken pathways, and pedestrian traffic lights without auditory signals—or to the social environment, whereby discriminating social attitudes can create social isolation and segregation. Alternatively, environments can be facilitatory and supportive, thus enabling people to conduct their everyday lives as they want and need to.

In addition to the three environmental dimensions, MOHO conceptualizes the environment in terms of three levels of context in which people live: "immediate contexts such as home, work, and school; local contexts such as the neighborhood and community; and global societal contexts" (Fisher et al. 2017, p. 93). The whole dynamic system of person-in-context is emphasized when each environmental dimension (physical, social, and occupational) mapped onto these three levels of context (immediate, local, and global). Each level interacts with the others and with the person embedded within them, and the three environmental dimensions interact with each other and with the levels. Fisher et al. noted that culture is present within every level of this complex system. They defined culture as "the beliefs and perceptions, values and norms, customs and behaviors that are shared by a group or society and are passed from one generation to the next through both formal and informal education" (p. 99). Culture pervades the whole dynamic system, underpinning the way all three levels of the environmental context are organized, as well is being internalized by the person.

In summary, the fifth edition of MOHO presents human occupation as a dynamic whole that comprises the transaction among people's volition, habituation, and performance and a multilayered environmental context. It provides a clear structure for understanding and navigating the complexity of human occupation. The personal and environmental elements provide a focus for analysis of the transactional occupational whole and an understanding of how occupation is selected, organized, and undertaken. Before discussing the use of MOHO in practice, we present three additional theoretical perspectives central to MOHO: (1) dimensions of doing, (2) a narrative approach to the lifespan, and (3) pathways of change in MOHO.

Dimensions of Doing

All the elements—those internal to the person, such as volition, habituation, and performance capacity, and those of the environment in which people live—influence what people do and how they do it. MOHO identifies the following three dimensions of doing: occupational participation, occupational performance, and skill. First, de las Heras de Pablo et al. (2017) stated that "*occupational participation* defines what we do in the broadest sense ... [and] describes our engagement in the broadest categories of work (study), play, and the activities of daily living that undergird everyday life" (p. 107). Occupational participation includes performance and its subjective experience and has both personal and social significance. The authors emphasized that use of the concept of participation in MOHO aligns with the *International Classification of Functioning, Disability and Health (ICF)* and the Occupational Therapy Practice Framework (OTPF). Participation in occupation requires feeling, thinking, and acting to different degrees, depending on the demands of what is being undertaken, the specific context, and the performance capacities, volition, and performance of the person. The second dimension of doing is *occupational performance*, which "comprises discrete acts, or units of doing, that are performed" (p. 107). Using Nelson's (1988) concepts of occupational form and performance, occupational performance involves engaging in an occupational form (i.e., performing an occupational form). Occupational performance can refer to the whole act being performed and the steps that are involved. De las Heras de Pablo et al. (2017) gave the example of cycling, which also involves the steps of preparing the bike, deciding where to ride, perhaps finding someone to ride with, mounting the bike, and pedaling. Third, the *skill* dimension of doing refers to those skills that are required to perform the occupation. In MOHO, these are categorized as motor skills (related to moving self or objects), process skills (logically sequencing actions over time), and communication and interaction skills (conveying needs and intentions and acting with others). What people do and how they do it affects how they think and feel about themselves and contributes to both occupational identity and occupational competence.

A Narrative Aproach to the Lifespan

MOHO also emphasizes that human occupation changes over time as age and circumstances change and that it needs to be understood from a whole-of-life perspective. Drawing upon narrative theory, Melton et al. (2017) explained that "people conduct and draw meaning from life by locating themselves in unfolding narratives that integrate their past, present, and future selves" (p. 125). Lives have a temporal dimension and people have a biographical history that shapes their interpretations and behaviors in the present. They also think, feel, and act in the present according to their goals and aspirations for the future.

Melton et al. (2017) presented two elements of narrative, plot and metaphor, that people use to synthesize their lives and create meaning for their experiences. *Plot* gives narrative its structure and provides the temporal linking of separate events into an integrated whole. Common examples of plots that could characterize a person's life narrative are tragic plots (with a steep downward turn) and melodramatic plots (with a series of ups and downs). Narratives have an overall shape—for example, they might be largely progressive (upward), regressive (downward), or stable (slight ups and downs around a middle point)—and the overall narrative shape of a person's life will influence their interpretation of individual events. For example, if a person's life narrative is generally progressive or stable, they are more likely to interpret a particular event positively than someone with a regressive shape to their life narrative. Thus events that are temporally separated (past and present) and aspirations for and expectations of the future can be bound together into a meaningful whole.

Metaphor is a figure of speech in which a familiar object or phenomenon is substituted for something else. Metaphors are useful for conveying a depth of meaning that would be difficult to express using description alone. For example, severe depression could be described using the metaphor of an ominous, looming dark cloud. Often, metaphors carry meanings that relate to the broader culture or society and therefore become imbued with shared meanings. For example, in current times, if something was described as pandemic, most people would share in the fear and image of dramatic, widespread and sweeping effects and changes. Metaphors can be used to pinpoint problems and imply solutions. Melton et al. (2017) gave the examples of using metaphors of momentum to suggest solutions that might involve changing pace or direction and metaphors of entrapment that imply the need for freedom and escape.

Using the concept of a narrative organization of life, Melton et al. (2017) used the term *occupational narrative* to refer to the story of how people's "volition, habituation, performance capacity, and environment interact over time" (p. 123) to shape what they do with their lives. People use occupational narratives to integrate the disparate elements of their life, such as what they do and experience. These narratives guide their occupational identity and sense of occupational competence.

The concept of occupational narrative emphasizes the temporal nature of human occupation. MOHO presents human occupation as a complex phenomenon with a range of dimensions. It results from the complex interactions over time between unique individuals—with their own particular motivations, interests, and values (volition); habits, routines, and internalized roles (habituation); and capabilities and experiences of themselves and their lives (performance capacity and the lived experience)—and their environments. These interactions can be relatively stable or marked by upward or downward trends over time.

Pathways of Change in MOHO

Throughout people's lives, they are constantly changing and developing. In the language of dynamic systems theory, the whole person-in-environment system constantly adapts to its changing situation by reorganizing when required to fulfill its goals and purposes. This means that its various elements—volition, habituation, performance, and environment—continually change and reorganize to create new states of equilibrium. Because the person-in-environment system is a dynamic whole, change in any component will promote changes in the other components and their unique configuration. Consequently, any of the four elements can provide the starting point for change.

When volition provides the initial pathway, a person's sense of agency, values, and interests can guide the selection of occupations. Because the person will be motivated to engage in those occupations, their actions will lead to a change in their patterns of engagement and the possible development of new roles (*habituation*). As their occupational engagement becomes more organized and consistent, they are likely to become more competent and experience their occupational participation positively (*performance capacity and the lived body*) and they will seek environments that afford such occupational engagement (*environment*). This illustrates that a change in volition will result in alteration in the whole system.

While volition and motivation might appear to be an obvious place to start, for people who enjoy order, ritual, and routine, habituation might form the better initial pathway to change. Similarly, performance might best provide the initial pathway for those who value and delight in their ability to carry out occupations. Being able to see improvement in their performance compared with baseline measurements might be the most engaging for them. And, finally, the environment might form the most appropriate initial pathway for change for some people. Changing the environment might include strategies such as home modifications, provision of equipment or personal assistance, as well as advocating for changes at the municipal and government levels through accessible transport, universal design, community activities and facilities, inclusive education, equitable distribution of resources, and so forth. People can more easily perform their occupations in environments that match their capacities.

Change is understood as having three stages on a continuum from exploration, to competence, and then to achievement. First, through exploration of occupations, people can discover and affirm their interests, preferences, capabilities, and potential effects on their relationships and lifestyles. Second, as people settle into undertaking new occupations and different ways of doing them, achieving consistent and adequate performance becomes a focus. New skills are developed, old skills are refined, and new habits and routines may be acquired. As competency builds, so too does self-efficacy. Third, the achievement stage of change involves integration of the new occupations and habits into a person's whole life. Occupational identity is reshaped, and established roles are altered to encompass the new area of occupational participation. People may move backward and forward between these three stages until new meaningful areas of occupational participation are established.

Having covered the main concepts in MOHO—the four elements of volition, habituation, performance capacity and the lived body, and environment, along with their components—we now turn to using the model in practice. As we discussed in Chapter 1, models aim to guide reasoning and decision-making. MOHO provides substantial resources for use in practice. We provide a brief overview of its approach to resourcing practice both conceptually and with assessments, and we encourage readers to access the details in the vast range of publications that are available. After this brief overview of using MOHO in practice, we discuss the extensive development of the model from a historical perspective over more than four decades.

Use of the Model in Practice

Using MOHO in practice comprises a seven-step therapeutic reasoning process that is client centered and theory driven (see Table 6.2). The term *therapeutic reasoning* is used instead of *clinical reasoning* to avoid biomedical connotations associated with the latter term. The first step is *generating theory-driven questions to inform nonstandardized assessment*. To use MOHO in practice, occupational therapists need to have a good understanding of the MOHO theory. The major concepts in MOHO theory are volition, habituation, performance capacity and the lived body, occupational participation, occupational performance, skills, environment, occupational identity, and occupational competence. Questions can be developed for each of these theoretical concepts. Forsyth (2017) provides extensive tables of questions for each concept in MOHO to guide therapeutic reasoning, and readers are referred to them for detailed examples of theory-driven questions. The second step is *administering standardized assessment*. A range of standardized assessments have been developed for MOHO and guidance for choosing them is discussed in the MOHO text. The third step is *creating an occupational formulation* of the client's situation. An occupational formulation brings together all the information obtained through assessment, and the occupational therapist reflects on it using the profession's knowledge base, the theoretical principles of MOHO, and their own reasoning. The fourth step is *identifying occupational changes*. These may relate to personal causation, values, interests, habits, roles, skills, and the social and physical environments, and this step involves identifying the changes that are desired and needed. The fifth step is developing measurable *goals*. These aim to address the occupational changes identified and that are measurable. Forsyth identified four elements of measurable goals: (1) occupational change, in which the nature of the occupational change is specified, including what the client will do to demonstrate that it has been achieved; (2) setting, or outlining where the intervention will be undertaken, such as the client's home or community, or a hospital or care facility; (3) degree, or specifying how the client will engage, such as independently, or with physical support or verbal cueing; and (4) the time frame in which it will be undertaken. The sixth step is *implementing intervention*. Forsyth emphasizes that the primary role of occupational therapists is to actively engage clients in meaningful occupations. This will improve their occupational identity and competence, thus improving their health and well-being. The seventh and final step is *assessing outcomes of intervention*. This involves evaluating the attainment of the measurable goals and may include repeating standardized assessments to determine the extent of change since baseline measurements.

MOHO has a suite of assessment tools to support using the model in practice. Each tool addresses a different constellation of concepts, and they range from the broad Model of Human Occupation Screening Tool and the Occupational Self-Assessment to assessments that address specific concepts, such as Interest Checklist, Role Checklist, and Vocational Questionnaire. Table 6.3 provides an overview of tools and the concepts they assess. Box 6.1 provides a case

---

TABLE 6.2 ■ **Therapeutic reasoning process**

1. Generating theory-driven questions to inform nonstandardized assessment
2. Administering standardized assessment
3. Creating an occupational formulation
4. Identifying occupational changes
5. Developing measurable goals
6. Implementing intervention
7. Assessing outcomes of intervention

TABLE 6.3 ■ MOHO Assessments

Concepts addressed by the assessment	Occupational adaptation		Volition			Habituation		Skills			Performance	Participation	Environment	
Assessment	Identity	Competence	Personal causation	Values	Interests	Roles	Habits	Motor	Process	Communication/Interaction			Physical	Social
Assessment of communication and interaction skills	×									×				
Assessment of motor and process skills		×						×	×					
Assessment of occupational functioning	×	×	×	×	×	×	×	×						
Child occupational self-assessment	×	×	×	×	×	×	×		×			×	×	
Interest checklist	×				×									
Model of Human Occupation screening tool	×	×	×	×	×	×	×	×	×	×	×	×	×	×
NIH activity record	×	×	×	×	×	×	×		×					
Occupational circumstances assessment—interview and rating scale	×	×	×	×	×	×	×		×					
Occupational performance history interview II	×	×	×	×	×	×	×	×						
Occupational questionnaire	×	×	×	×	×	×					×			
Occupational self-assessment	×	×	×	×	×	×	×	×		×		×	×	×

Assessment							
Occupational therapy psychosocial assessment of learning	X	X	X	X	X			X
Pediatric interest profile	X	X	X	X			
Pediatric volitional questionnaire	X	X	X	X			
Role checklist	X	X	X				
School setting interview	X	X					
Short child occupational profile	X	X	X	X	X	X	X
Volitional questionnaire	X	X					
Worker role interview	X	X	X	X	X		
Work environment impact scale	X	X					

NIH, National Institutes of Health.
Adapted from Kielhofner 2008, pp. 160–161.

BOX 6.1 ■ Case Illustration

Melany is an occupational therapist who works in a correctional center. Her role is to promote social and work reintegration for men who have been incarcerated in a low-risk unit. Paul is a 45-year-old inmate who was sent to jail one year ago, after two people died as a result of an accident he caused when driving under the influence of alcohol. Paul is married and has two adolescent children. Before the accident he worked as an electrician, but he had family difficulties and problems at work because of his drinking habits. During the initial interview and looking through the lens of MOHO, Melany realized Paul narrated his life as a melodramatic plot. Paul's father abandoned his family when he was 10 years old, after which his mother became an alcoholic. In primary school, he had excellent support from teachers and achieved good academic results. However his life became complicated in high school when he started to display behavioral difficulties, such as having fights with classmates, consuming alcohol, and taking drugs.

After assessing Paul, Melany identified that he especially valued his roles of father and husband. Consequently, he wanted to participate in the workshops available at the correctional center in the hope of being able to provide financial support to his family. But Melany also observed that Paul's personal causation had been affected by his incarceration; that is, he thought he did not deserve another opportunity because he felt "guilty for being a murderer" and he was embarrassed by his new role of "prisoner." Therefore he did not feel he should participate in the workshops that were offered, such as pottery or carpentry, even though he knew he would find them interesting. Assessment of Paul's objective performance capacity revealed that he did not have any structural or functional difficulties. In terms of his subjective performance, he felt his background as an electrician would not give him the skills he would need for carpentry. Therefore Melanie could see that, while his physical capacities would be well matched to carpentry and the habits he formed as an electrician would be an advantage, his perception of his own limited capabilities and effectiveness made him uncertain and he needed reassurance and encouragement.

As part of his social environment, Melany knew she could be a positive influence in his life. She planned steps to promote the pathways of change and encouraged Paul to *explore* the workshops and try different occupations. After initially being tentative, Paul appeared very engaged while completing tasks at the carpentry workshop and was motivated to continue. The following week, to progress to the next step of change, *competence*, Melany organized a member of the workshop to provide specific training to Paul. Paul attended the workshops regularly, and after three years he had become a skilled carpenter, with well-entrenched habits of occupational performance, habits of routine, and habits of style. As he was soon to be released from jail and to help him progress to the third stage of change, *achievement*, Melany decided to commence an intervention with his social environment. She connected with a community health organization to ensure that Paul would receive ongoing mental health services and family counseling and would support his social reintegration as he ventured into the world outside of prison. To support his valued roles of father and husband, with his permission she contacted his family to help them prepare for his reentrance into family life. To support his adoption of the worker role again, Melany identified several companies that might employ Paul. By comparing his current capacities and sense of self with her baseline assessments, she was able to evaluate the effectiveness of her intervention while he had been in prison. She also planned to continue to monitor his situation for a time after his release to support him as he took up his valued social roles again.

---

illustration of Melanie, an occupational therapist working with Paul in a correctional center to help him reestablish his roles.

Historical Description of the Model's Development

MOHO is an occupational therapy model that has had a very long publication history. According to Kielhofner (2008), MOHO was first published in 1980 in a series of four articles in the *American Journal of Occupational Therapy*. He described the model as "the product of three occupational therapy practitioners attempting to articulate concepts that guided their practice" (Kielhofner 2008, p. 1). As a single volume, MOHO has been published in five editions, commencing in 1985 and spanning the intervening decades to 2017 (the last one to be edited by Kielhofner was 2008). It is a conceptual model that has influenced occupational therapy theory and practice over possibly the most sustained period of the profession's history.

MOHO was developed at a time when occupational therapy was very influenced by the ideas of the biomedical model of health. According to Madigan and Parent (1985), Mary Reilly, from the University of Southern California (USC), had been cautioning occupational therapy since the late 1950s that its alignment with medicine was too narrowing. Reilly's argument had been that medicine's focus was on the prevention and reduction of disease and illness, whereas occupational therapy dealt with the process of helping people adapt their lives to develop and preserve life satisfaction "through work and social development" (Madigan and Parent 1985, p. vii). Reilly's theory of occupational behavior guided research and teaching at USC for a number of decades and was an important influence in the development of MOHO.

In 1985, Madigan and Parent explained that the MOHO publication was "the latest compilation of many persons' efforts to build and apply a theory unique to occupational therapy" (Madigan and Parent 1985, p. vii). At that time, Kielhofner explained the need for a model by placing this need in the context of the extensive development of concepts that occurred in the occupational behavior tradition. He stated, "Since the number of concepts grew to be large and somewhat cumbersome, it became necessary to develop models of practice which integrated these concepts into a workable format. The model of human occupation began as one such model which sought to build upon the existing occupational behavior tradition" (Kielhofner, cited in Madigan and Parent 1985, p. xviii).

It appears that, at the time of the 1985 publication, it was unclear whether Kielhofner's MOHO was "an extension and further evolution of occupational behavior theory" or whether it was a new direction in theory (Madigan and Parent 1985, p. ix). While it was clear that the model flowed logically from occupational behavior in terms of its major concepts of "role, interests, values, personal causation, intrinsic motivation, and environment, to name a few" (Madigan and Parent 1985, p. ix), Reed was cited as taking the position that MOHO was different from occupational behavior theory (although clearly developed from it). Over time, as the model has been further developed, its difference from occupational behavior theory has been clearly demonstrated.

In some ways the model has changed enormously over time, while its overall structure has remained similar. A major change is the way its basis in systems theory has been described over time. The language used to refer to the various parts of the system has changed across the five editions as the theoretical perspectives of systems theory changed. The first edition, in 1985, used open systems theory and labeled volition, habituation, and performance as *subsystems* that had a hierarchical relationship (with volition being at the top of the hierarchy). In the second edition, based on dynamic systems theory, volition, habituation, and performance were referred to as a hierarchy of *subcomponents* (explained later) and in the third (2002) and fourth (2008) editions, they are called *interrelated components* and are conceptualized as nonhierarchical and mutually influencing. In the fifth edition, four *elements* are identified as dynamically connected: volition, habituation, performance capacity and the lived body, and environment. (In the fifth edition, the clear distinction between person and environment that was evident in the first four editions is broken down and environment is presented as just one of four elements in the system.)

When explaining the systems basis of the model in the first four editions, Kielhofner contrasted it with a mechanistic perspective. Kielhofner (2002) explained in the third edition that the model had originally been developed in response to the profession's previous alignment with medicine, with its mechanistic understanding of health (which Mary Reilly had criticized as creating too narrow a focus in the profession). MOHO was originally developed when biomedicine was the dominant perspective in health. However, as explained in the introduction to this book, the adoption of systems theory in the area of health allowed for a broader understanding in Western countries of the factors that affect an individual's health. MOHO was developed at a time when a systems approach was being proposed for understanding health (e.g., by Engels).

The first two editions of MOHO explained in detail various aspects of systems theory as the basis for its understanding of human occupation. In the first edition the model was presented as based on *open systems theory*. In that edition Kielhofner (1985) contrasted open and closed systems theory by showing that closed systems (e.g., machines) wear down (entropy) while open systems, which are open to receive energy from the outside, have the capacity to build up and become more complex (negative entropy). Open systems are conceptualized as having subsystems that are organized in a hierarchical relationship. In such a hierarchy, the higher subsystems command the lower subsystems and the lower ones constrain the higher ones. In the first edition of MOHO, volition, habituation, and performance were conceptualized as subsystems that were arranged in a hierarchical relationship. For example, volition was considered the highest subsystem and was thought to command the lower ones, but also be constrained by them. Similarly, habituation (in the middle of the hierarchy) is commanded by volition and constrained by performance.

The second edition of MOHO is based on *dynamic systems theory*. A major difference between dynamic and open systems theory is that, in dynamic systems, the organism is considered to have the capacity to reorganize itself. The way systems maintain themselves in optimal conditions is referred to as their "steady state" (Kielhofner 1985, p. 7). In open systems theory, while systems are able to increase in complexity when they deviate from their steady state, they maintain their essential structure. However dynamic systems theory assumes that organisms are able to reorganize themselves and become more complex. Prigogine and Stengers (1984), in their book *Order out of Chaos*, used the example of water flowing in a stream to illustrate the capacity for systems to reorganize when their steady state is disrupted. As water flows over rocks, it becomes increasingly destabilized and chaotic (splashes, etc.). However, as its steady state becomes more and more disturbed, it can reorganize itself—for example, into a whirlpool, which is organized differently from the currents in the original stream.

Consistent with this change from open systems theory to dynamic systems theory, the relationship between the subsystems/elements of MOHO (volition, habituation, and performance) in the second edition were no longer considered a hierarchy but a *heterarchy*. As Kielhofner (1995) explained, "The concept of heterarchy recognizes that systems arrange themselves according to the demands of situations in which they are performing, not according to a preordained or fixed structure" (p. 34).

In the second edition of MOHO, the concept of heterarchy was applied through the assumption of a "dynamical assembly of behavior" (Kielhofner 1995, p. 14). When using a mechanistic metaphor (e.g., body-as-machine metaphor in biomedicine), the assumption is that "structure causes function" (e.g., the heart functions as a pump because of its structure). When applied to behavior, this suggests that the behavior of an organism can be predicted according to its structure. However, where a machine metaphor breaks down is that the structure of humans is unable to explain their *potential* for behavior and how they select from all possible behaviors available to them. As Kielhofner (1995) stated, "Humans perform in an almost infinite variety of emotional, cognitive, and physical circumstances" (p. 15) and he proposed that, because humans can assemble their behavior differently as circumstances demand, no two performances of the same activity will be exactly the same. Just as the water flowing across rocks can reorganize itself to suit the surroundings, so too do humans engage in "self-organization" through occupation. As Kielhofner (1995) stated, "When we work, play, and perform the tasks of daily life, we are not merely engaging in occupational behavior, we are organizing ourselves. We use our bodies and minds in the contexts of occupations, organizing them accordingly. We create our motor abilities, our self-concepts, [and] social identities in our occupations. Occupational behaviour is self-making." (p. 22.)

In the third and fourth editions, a systems perspective is discussed as a general concept (rather than being explained in detail, as in the first two editions) and is contrasted with a mechanistic perspective. This contrast illustrates the danger of occupational therapy practice being dominated by a reductionistic, biomedical perspective and losing sight of its occupation-based perspective. The third edition of MOHO contrasts machines and robots (representing closed systems without making that explicit) with the concepts underpinning MOHO (which belong to dynamic systems theory). The concepts of heterarchy and emergence are discussed in both the third and fourth editions and control parameter is discussed in the fourth edition. We explain these three concepts in the paragraphs that follow.

Heterarchy can be contrasted with hierarchy. Whereas a hierarchical structure is one in which the higher levels command the lower levels and the lower levels constrain the higher levels, heterarchy assumes a nonhierarchical organization in which the components function according to the needs of the whole. That is, components contribute to the whole according to their capacities, and the relationship between different components is reorganized according to the requirements of the whole. In relation to MOHO, this means the four elements—volition, habituation, performance, and environment—are assembled (or called upon) according to the occupational requirements in the situation. Whenever a person engages in occupation in a particular context, all four elements are uniquely combined to achieve the goal. *Emergence* is defined as "the principle that complex actions, thoughts, and feelings spontaneously arise out of the interactions of several components" (Kielhofner 2008, p. 25). What a person thinks or feels is not predetermined but *emerges* from the combination of volition, habituation, performance, and environment (which has been uniquely assembled for each situation). While some components support and others constrain particular behaviors, it is the summation of their contributions to the whole that results in the emergence of certain behaviors, thoughts, and feelings. A *control parameter* is any factor that changes the whole dynamic when it changes. For example, not all changes in aspects of volition, habituation, performance, and the environment will change the dynamic assemblage, but when a "critical change" occurs, it results in a "different emergent behaviour" (p. 26). This means a change in any of volition, habituation, performance, and/or the environment "can result in a change in the thoughts, feelings, and doing that make up one's occupation" (p. 26), which will then change the response required.

The fifth edition of MOHO (Taylor 2017) builds on this dynamic systems theory approach and presents the four elements—volition, habituation, performance, and environment—together as a transactional whole as if in an orbit around the model itself. While the preceding four editions were based on various forms of systems theory, the fifth edition is explicitly based on a dynamic systems theory understanding of how occupation occurs. A historical view of MOHO reflects the general conceptual journey of occupational therapy itself. While MOHO was initially developed to organize the concepts embedded in the Occupational Behaviour approach, and its opposition to a narrow biomedical approach (as seen in the occupational performance models), it commenced with and maintained a clear distinction between person and environment until the fifth edition. Occupational therapy has also largely maintained a clear separation between person and environment while increasingly emphasizing the situatedness of people in their environments. While MOHO is the only model that has consistently highlighted systems theory for understanding the various aspects of human occupation, its five editions show a gradual progression toward a transactional perspective of people-in-their-environment, which is consistent with a trend in occupational therapy more broadly.

Memory Aid

See Box 6.2.

BOX 6.2 ■ Memory Aid

To develop an occupational formulation, review the information you have collected and reflect on questions such as these. You can also use these kinds of questions to guide the information you collect.

Occupational identity: As an occupational being, what is this person's sense of who they are, have been, and will/want to be in the future?

Occupational competence: How well has this person maintained a pattern of occupational engagement and participation that is consistent with their sense of occupational identity?

Participation: In what ways does this person participate (or want to participate) in their sociocultural context through work, play, and activities of daily living in response to their needs/wants and society's expectations?

Performance: What occupational forms/tasks is this person able/unable to do in the areas of work, play, and activities of daily living?

Skills: How well does this person's motor, process, and/or communication/interaction skills match what they want/need to do?

Volition: What are this person's motivations, values, and interests? To what degree do they feel able to influence their occupations, circumstances, and environment?

Habituation: What roles does the person need/want to fulfill? How well do their habits support their ability to engage in occupations and roles in their particular environment?

Performance capacity and the lived body: How do this person's body systems support performance? How do they experience engagement in occupation? What is this person's embodied experience of acting in the world?

Environment: How does the environment impact this person's occupational engagement (opportunities and resources that it provides, demands and constraints that it imposes) at the immediate, local, and global levels?

What initial pathway to change might be most effective in promoting exploration for the person?

Adapted from Forsyth K. Therapeutic reasoning: planning, implementing and evaluating the outcomes of therapy. In: Taylor RR, ed. *Kielhofner's Model of Human Occupation: Theory and Application.* 5th ed. Wolters Kluwer; 2017:159–172.

Conclusion

MOHO is the occupational therapy model of practice with the longest continuous progress, being updated and developed for more than four decades to date. It was first created to provide organization to the many concepts associated with the Occupational Behaviour tradition. The structure of the model is based on systems theory. Over time, this has developed from Open Systems theory to Dynamic Systems theory. Originally, MOHO focused on the person as a system comprising the subsystems/elements of volition, habituation, and performance with their various components. The person and their environment were viewed as separate entities. However, consistent with the current trend in occupational therapy models, the fifth edition of MOHO conceptualizes the environment as *part* of the dynamic system. Consequently, the four elements of volition, habituation, performance, and environment comprise an integrated and dynamic whole, which can reorganize itself to adapt to current circumstances. This means people must always be considered within the real-life contexts in which they live. They cannot be understood separately from their immediate context of home, work, school, and, if relevant, treatment facility, as well as their local and global contexts. What they think, feel, and do and the routines they develop and roles they adopt are always shaped by their context, just as these things also shape those contexts. To understand that the environment is part of the dynamic system, the fifth edition of MOHO places greater emphasis on the environment and its various components than earlier editions of the model.

A unique feature of MOHO is the substantial development of assessment tools. No other model of practice has developed tools to the same extent. Consistent with the model's focus on subjective experience, these assessments use observation, self-report, and interview. The model also provides a client-centered and theory-driven process to follow in practice.

References

De las Heras de Pablo CG, Fan CW, Kielhofner G. Dimensions of doing. In: Taylor RR, ed. *Kielhofner's Model of Human Occupation: Theory and Application.* 5th ed. Wolters Kluwer; 2017:107–122.

Fisher G, Parkinson S, Haglund L. The environment and human occupation. In: Taylor RR, ed. *Kielhofner's Model of Human Occupation: Theory and Application.* 5th ed. Wolters Kluwer; 2017:91–106.

Forsyth K. Therapeutic reasoning: planning, implementing and evaluating the outcomes of therapy. In: Taylor RR, ed. K*ielhofner's Model of Human Occupation: Theory and Application.* 5th ed. Wolters Kluwer; 2017:159–172.

Kielhofner G. A model of human occupation: Theory and application. 4th ed. Lippincott Williams & Wilkins; 2008.

Lee SW, Kielhofner G. Volition. In: Taylor RR, ed. *Kielhofner's Model of Human Occupation: Theory and Application.* 5th ed. Wolters Kluwer; 2017a:38–56.

Lee SW, Kielhofner G. Habituation: patterns of daily occupation. In: Taylor RR, ed. *Kielhofner's Model of Human Occupation: Theory and Application.* 5th ed. Wolters Kluwer; 2017b:57–73.

Madigan MJ, Parent LH. Preface. In: Kielhofner G, ed. A model of human occupation: Theory and application. 4th ed. Lippincott Williams & Wilkins; 1985:vi–ix.

Melton J, Holzmueller RP, Keponen R, Nyggard L, Munger K, Kielhofner G. Crafting occupational life. In: Taylor RR, ed. *Kielhofner's Model of Human Occupation: Theory and Application.* 5th ed. Wolters Kluwer; 2017:123–139.

Nakamura J, Csikszentmihalyi M. The concept of flow. In: *Flow and the Foundations of Positive Psychology.* Springer; 2014:239–263.

Nelson DL. Occupation: form and performance. *Am J Occup Ther.* 1988 Oct;42(10):633–641. doi:10.5014/ajot.42.10.633

O'Brien JC, Kielhofner G. The interaction between the person and the environment. In: Taylor RR, ed. *Kielhofner's Model of Human Occupation: Theory and Application.* 5th ed. Wolters Kluwer; 2017:24–37.

Taylor RR, Kielhofner G. Introduction to the Model of Human Occupation. In: Taylor RR, ed. *Kielhofner's Model of Human Occupation: Theory and Application.* 5th ed. Wolters Kluwer; 2017:3–10.

Tham K, Erickson A, Fallaphour M, Taylor RR, Kielhofner G. Performance capacity and the lived body. In: Taylor RR, ed. *Kielhofner's Model of Human Occupation: Theory and Application.* 5th ed. Wolters Kluwer; 2017:74–90.

Yamada T, Taylor RR, Kielhofner G. The person-specific concepts of human occupation. In: RR Taylor RR, ed. *Kielhofner's Model of Human Occupation: Theory and Application.* 5th ed. Wolters Kluwer; 2017:11–23.

Zola IK. *Missing Pieces: A Chronicle of Living with a Disability.* Temple University Press; 1982.

CHAPTER 7

The Canadian Model of Occupational Participation (CanMOP)

CHAPTER CONTENTS

The Canadian Model of Occupational Participation: Major Concepts and Definitions   136

Collaborative Relationship-Focused Occupational Therapy: Major Concepts and Definitions   142

Canadian Occupational Therapy Inter-relational Practice Process Framework: Major Concepts and Definitions   146

Historical Description of the Canadian Guidelines' Development   150

Memory Aid   154

Major Works   155

Summary   155

References   156

In 2022 the Canadian Association of Occupational Therapists (CAOT) published the book Promoting Occupational Participation: Collaborative Relationship-Focused Occupational Therapy (Promoting Occupational Participation) as part of its 10th Canadian Occupational Therapy guidelines. This book is the most recent in a series of books designed to address the question "what do occupational therapists do?" In answer to this question, it proposes that "occupational therapists are focused on helping people do the things they need to do and want to do, with the people and in the places that are important to them. Occupational Therapists work collaboratively with individuals and collectives (families, groups, communities, and populations) to support people to live the lives they consider to be good." (Egan and Restall 2022, p. 75). In helping to guide occupational therapists to achieve this, the book presents three types of theoretical guidelines: "a Model, Approach, and Framework for Occupational Therapy" (p. 71). In this chapter we present these three: the Canadian Model of Occupational Participation, the Collaborative Relationship-Focused Occupational Therapy approach, and the Canadian Occupational Therapy Inter-Relational Practice Process Framework. Pervading these three is an awareness of the vast diversity of people's experiences, particularly in relation to sociocultural diversity and the colonial history that has contributed to the experiences of First Nations people.

The Canadian Model of Occupational Participation: Major Concepts and Definitions

The *Canadian Model of Occupational Participation* (CanMOP) aims to provide guidance to occupational therapists "in their reflection, reasoning, and analysis about occupational participation"

(Egan and Restall 2022, p. 75). Occupational participation is defined as "*having access to, initiating, and sustaining valued occupations within meaningful relationships and contexts*" (p. 75, italics in original). In promoting occupational participation, occupational therapists also consider both occupational performance, which involves choosing, organizing, and performing meaningful occupations, and occupational engagement, which refers to performance "in the moment" (p. 76). Egan and Restall emphasized that focusing on occupational participation enables occupational therapists to "look beyond occupational performance" (p. 76). This reference to occupational performance is important because the previous Canadian models had long centered on that concept, whereas the notion of occupational participation includes the broader concern for being part of meaningful occupations. Through their core focus on occupational participation, occupational therapists "are concerned with helping people gain access to, initiate, and sustain occupations they need to or wish to pursue, how, where, when, and with whom they wish to pursue them" (p. 76). The model also makes it clear that occupational participation must be considered for both individuals and collectives (i.e., families, groups, communities, and populations).

Fig. 7.1 provides a diagrammatic representation of the main components of the CanMOP. The core of the model is occupational participation and the model presents two "central considerations" (p. 77) of occupational therapy, with each surrounded by important influences on it. The first central consideration is meaning and purpose, which is influenced by history and relationships. The second central consideration is occupational possibilities, which is shaped by context at the micro, meso, and macro levels.

Regarding the first central consideration of *meaning and purpose*, the model emphasizes that the meaning and purpose of occupational participation is specific to individuals and collectives. Meaning needs to be understood from the perspective of those individuals and collectives, rather than from that of the occupational therapist working with them. Consequently, occupational therapists are cautioned to be vigilant regarding not imposing their own assumptions about the meaning of occupation and are urged to be aware of their own perspectives and those of the dominant culture. Doing this will create an openness to the views and values of those with whom they are working.

An occupational therapist's understanding of the purpose of occupational participation should be guided by an individual's or a collective's perspective regarding their four basic needs of survival

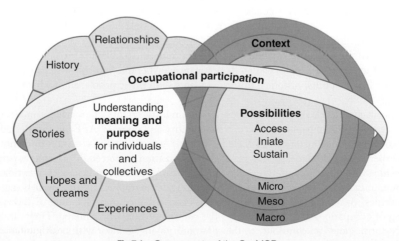

Fig 7.1   Components of the CanMOP.

and safety, autonomy, relatedness, and competence. First, Egan and Restall (2022) used the work of Maslow to explain that adequate survival and safety drives much behavior. In addition, it is important to understand that, from the perspective of Indigenous peoples, the survival needs of an individual and the physical, emotional, cognitive, and spiritual needs of the community are intertwined. Therefore, understanding any individual's impetus for survival and safety must include their obligations to the community (including ancestors and descendants). Next, Egan and Restall linked the other three basic needs of autonomy, relatedness, and competence to self-determination theory. A sense of *autonomy* occurs when a person feels their actions are consistent with their own values and community standards. *Relatedness* involves a sense of being connected with, supporting, and being supported by others. A sense of *competence* occurs when a person feels they have been effective in occupations that are important to them.

Relationships and *history* are identified as the context that shapes meaning and purpose, represented by the surrounding diamond shape in the diagram. Relationships play a central role in shaping the meaning and purpose of occupational participation. Individuals and collectives are part of a rich network of relationships, in which they "relate to each other, their physical environments, histories, ancestors, cultures, knowledges, social, political, and economic structures, and the natural world" (p. 79). Relationships often provide the fundamental purpose for engaging in occupation. Egan and Restall (2022) gave the example of a range of reasons for engaging in the occupation of fishing. It might be done for the varying purposes of contributing to the family's or community's food supply, communing with nature, continuing an ancestral occupation, improving a skill, spending time with friends, and sharing an occupation with children and grandchildren. The relationships within which people participate in an occupation shape why, what, and how it is done. Both time and relationships play a role in determining the meaning of occupation for individuals and collectives. As Egan and Restall stated, "past, present, and future hoped-for occupational participation always involves specific others, even when those others are present only in memory and imagination" (p. 79).

The notion of history is explored at both an individual and collective level. At an individual level, the CanMOP uses the Life Course perspective to place a person's life within its temporal context, deepening understanding of how the meaning and purpose of occupational participation are influenced by aspects of that life. The Life Course perspective has five principles: (1) lifelong development, which acknowledges that life unfolds over time and that past experiences influence the present; (2) historical time and place, which emphasizes that people's lives are shaped by the historical times and geographical contexts in which they live; (3) timing in lives, which stresses that the impact of life events depends on when they occur in a person's life, with earlier events affecting later experiences; (4) linked lives, in which people are understood to exist within networks of relationships with others; and (5) agency, whereby people are seen to be able to take action within the context of the opportunities and constraints afforded by their situation. Taken together, these principles can guide occupational therapists to consider people as agentic beings who live in specific historical times and places with other people, all of which shape their experiences of life.

At a collective level, the CanMOP uses a community history approach to understand the experiences of groups of people with a common identity and purpose. As Egan and Restall (2022) explained, community histories can include "historic experiences of cohesion and thriving, as well as experiences of trauma, such as genocide, colonization, or forced displacement; patterns of relationships with governments and various adjacent communities; and changes over time within the community related to size, geographic location, demographics, health, well-being, values, and priorities" (p. 80). Such community histories can enhance understanding of the value and meaning of occupations and the challenges the community has encountered. They can assist in setting priorities and can contribute to the community's engagement with health and social care providers.

The second essential consideration is *occupational possibilities* to access, initiate, and sustain participation in occupation. The background to this essential consideration is context, explored at the micro, meso, and macro levels. According to Egan and Restall (2022), occupational therapists are ready to engage with this second essential consideration once they have gained a good understanding of the meaning and purpose of an individual's or a collective's occupation. They used the definition of occupational possibilities provided by Laliberte Rudman (2010) as follows: "ways and types of doing that come to be viewed as ideal and possible with a specific socio-historical context, and that come to be promoted and made available within that context" (p. 55). Thus the notion of occupational possibilities emphasizes that context powerfully determines expectations, barriers, and affordances regarding occupational participation. Egan and Restall emphasized that consideration of occupational possibilities should be undertaken collaboratively. They presented occupational therapists as experts in expanding occupational possibilities by (1) addressing unexamined assumptions about what certain people who have differences in body structures and functions and social identities can and should do; and (2) collaboratively identifying and supporting needed changes to contexts at the micro, meso, and macro levels.

Expanding occupational possibilities requires a deep understanding of the relationship between people and their contexts. This involves comprehending both the characteristics of the individual or collective and the nature of the context. At the individual level, this includes their physical, affective, and cognitive structures and functions, as well as their values, beliefs, sense of spirituality, and social identities. At the collective level, it refers to the values, beliefs, and inter-relationships of families and communities, their shared histories, and the resources they have available to them and how they use those resources.

When considering context, the CanMOP uses an adapted version of Bronfenbrenner's (2004) levels of systems. It uses the three levels of micro, meso, and macro contexts. First, the *micro* context includes people's direct interactions, such as those with family members, friends, teachers and peers from school, co-workers, and providers of health and social services, as well as direct interactions with the physical environment. For communities, the micro context also includes the interactions that members have with one another. Second, the *meso* context refers to the level of social systems, including organizations and their respective programs and neighborhood and community infrastructure systems such as the built environment. At this level of context, occupational participation is affected by factors that are largely beyond the control of individuals. Examples include eligibility for services and what people must do to remain in programs, the availability and cost of travel, and the accessibility of built environments. Finally, the *macro* context level refers to the broader socioeconomic and political context and includes social and cultural values and beliefs that are reinforced by policy and legislation. The macro context regulates the meso context by determining what is allowed or prevented and what is funded. It greatly influences the work of occupational therapists and the occupational possibilities of the people with whom they work by creating a framework that designates what will be developed and provided by both public services and private enterprises. When reflecting on the service contexts in which occupational therapists work, Egan and Restall (2022) emphasized that these contexts frequently do not support the provision of collaborative relation-based practice. Therefore they proposed that, "ideally, while providing the best service possible under current circumstances, therapists work collaboratively to dismantle [macro-level] structures" (p. 82). To assist occupational therapists to analyze macro-level structures so that they can collectively work to dismantle them, *Promoting Occupational Participation* considers the broader sociopolitical context that powerfully shapes occupational possibilities. First, it discusses the social determinants of health, well-being, and occupation that lead to health inequities. Then it examines some distal determinants from a Canadian perspective (see Box 7.1).

BOX 7.1 ■ Social Determinants of Health and Health Inequalities

The World Health Organization (WHO) defines the social determinants of health as "the non-medical factors that influence health outcomes. They are the conditions in which people are born, grow, work, live, and age, and the wider set of forces and systems shaping the conditions of daily life" (WHO 2022). The examples provided by the WHO are income and social protection, education, unemployment and job insecurity, working life conditions, food insecurity, housing, basic amenities and the environment, early childhood development, social inclusion and nondiscrimination, structural conflict, and access to affordable health services of decent quality. Trentham et al. (2022) explained that these conditions have a greater influence on health and illness than biomedical care and strongly shape occupational possibilities. Variations in the social determinants of health result in health inequities. The social determinants of health are categorized into proximal determinants, intermediate determinants, and distal determinants, which can be equated with the micro, meso, and macro contexts in the CanMOP. The proximal determinants are social conditions that people interact with directly, while intermediate determinants extend beyond individuals and are often the foundations underpinning proximal determinants. "Distal determinants include historical, political, economic, and social structures of a society, ideologies and worldviews from which the intermediate and proximal determinants evolve" (Trentham et al. p. 34). Distal determinants are also referred to as structural determinants because they form the basis for the structures of society. They form the basis for systematically advantaging and disadvantaging certain groups of people.

Referring to the Canadian context, Trentham et al. (2022) discussed three distal determinants that reinforce social hierarchies and entrench disadvantage and oppression: colonialism, neoliberalism, and climate change. First, Canada's colonial history (as with other countries with colonial histories) is marked by the systematic oppression of Indigenous peoples through genocide, land theft and displacement, destruction of culture and family networks, and loss of languages. A history of violence and criminalization has led to "ongoing structural violence that penetrates the everyday lives of Indigenous peoples today" (p. 39). Canada's colonial legacy does not only affect Indigenous peoples. Settlers also brought with them a culture of racism, sexism, and ableism. The ideal notion of a person was "a Western, Euro-white, able-bodied, working-aged, heterosexual male" (p. 39), and settler culture was organized to advantage people with these attributes. Consequently, people with characteristics varying from this ideal, such as people of color, women, people who are nonbinary and LGBTIQ+, older adults, and people who are not able-bodied, are seen as inferior and face systematic disadvantage. For example, people can be disabled by the structure of the built environment, transport, health, education, employment, and so forth.

Occupational therapists need to careful not to pathologize the effects of this historical trauma by only viewing health problems through a biomedical perspective, and instead to recognize the root causes of health inequalities.

Second, two key features of neoliberalism are market-based practices and individualism. In neoliberalism, freedom of economic markets is prioritized, aiming to optimize economic benefit and efficiencies. When applied to healthcare, welfare, and education, return on investment is prioritized over public good. This often leads to cuts in funding and reduction in services, resulting in increased inequities and failure to recognize other types of positive outcomes. When individual self-interest, independence, and responsibility are prioritized over interdependence and collective responsibility, success is generally determined by markers relating to individuals, with the health and well-being of communities often being overlooked. In a neoliberal service context, occupational therapists often work with individuals and focus on the level of micro contexts. However, Trentham et al. cautioned that, with such an individual focus, their work might center on adapting their clients to fit oppressive systems, rather than working collectively to dismantle such systems and promoting the development of equitable and just systems that uphold human rights. Trentham et al. summarized the impact of neoliberalism by saying that "Neoliberalism serves to perpetuate ablest and ageist understandings of disability as resulting from individual deficits rather than social barriers"; that it frames poverty as the result of people's choices and behaviors, rather than being due to systemic inequities; and that it "negates the pervasive impacts of colonisation on family's and children's everyday lives through shaping ahistorical, decontextualised services that focus on *deficits* particularly with respect to indigenous children" (p. 41).

Continued

BOX 7.1 ■ Social Determinants of Health and Health Inequalities—cont'd

Third, regarding the climate crisis, Trentham et al. (2022) explained that, while occupational therapists acknowledge the intricate and inseparable nature of people and their context, insufficient attention has been paid to connection to land. Lack of respect for the natural world is another legacy of colonialism and neoliberalism. While climate change affects everyone, it disproportionately affects those who are vulnerable and disadvantaged.

Trentham et al. (2022) proposed that acknowledgment and consideration of the social determinants of health, particularly the distal, structural determinants that pervade the organization of society, are important for both individual therapists and the profession of occupational therapy. At the broader level, educators, regulators, scholars, and professional association leaders need to consider issues such as ensuring representation of diverse groups, especially from those groups that have been historically marginalized, interrogating occupational therapy models, frameworks, processes, and practices for perpetuation of systematic disadvantage and oppression. They emphasize the importance of dialogue, collaboration, partnerships, and allyship in paving a way forward.

The CanMOP emphasizes that these three levels of context affect the possibilities for occupational participation by promoting and limiting possibilities for accessing, initiating, and sustaining occupation. As Egan and Restall (2022) stated, "critically examining the aspects of contexts that promote or limit occupational participation for individuals or collectives gives occupational therapists tools to seek opportunities to build on strengths, reduce barriers, and expand occupational possibilities" (p. 82). For each concept—access, initiate, and sustain—the CanMOP provides guidance to occupational therapists regarding how the micro, meso, and macro aspects of context can be inhibiting. We discuss this guidance in the paragraphs that follow.

First, occupational therapists can promote occupational participation by improving *access* to occupations at community and population levels. Factors that limit occupational possibilities can be both explicit and implicit, and occupational therapists can work to highlight these barriers to access and help organizations address them. Egan and Restall (2022) emphasized that such interventions aim to improve access for people in general, rather than for specific individuals, and gave examples of actions occupational therapists might take to improve accessibility. Interventions include asking people about the barriers to access they have experienced, advocating with municipal bodies to improve access to hiking trails and other aspects of the built environment, and intervening to reduce stigma, discrimination, and oppression in private and public spaces. In general, enhancing access involves addressing barriers at the meso and macro levels of context. Occupational therapists need to continue their vigilance about access because, while some improvements may be made at a specific time, other issues of access, particularly implicit factors such as social attitudes, can remain persistent barriers.

Second, people need to be able to *initiate* contextually meaningful occupation. Occupational participation often requires the initiation or reinitiation of valued occupation. Factors that impede initiation can be concrete or abstract. Concrete challenges can relate to cost, time, insufficient skill or confidence, and limited public services such as transport. An example of abstract challenges is social attitudes that reduce acceptance of new people. As Egan and Restall (2022) explained, "occupational therapists collaborate with an individual or collective to explore occupational possibilities, understand the occupations that people need and desire to participate in, and co-create plans to make initiation of participation in valued occupations possible" (pp. 83–84).

Third, people need to be able to *sustain* occupational participation over time. Factors that influence the ability to sustain occupation occur at micro, meso, and macro levels and can be explicit or implicit. Factors at all three levels are mutually influencing. For example, a child might not be able to sustain participation in sport because, at a micro level, their coach is unable to accommodate the child's needs and the child finds it too distressing to continue. However, this micro-level challenge may be a consequence of a larger meso-level issue pertaining to lack of training of coaches on different ways to facilitate the participation of children with disabilities. And this situation may relate to a macro-level problem of limited policies and funding to support such training. Occupational therapists can work at all these different levels. For example, they might work with the child to help enhance their resilience (micro level), work with the coach to build their skills in supporting disabled children to participate (meso level), and advocate at the macro level for appropriate policies and funding to support training.

In summary, the CanMOP is centered explicitly on occupational participation, whereby people have access to and can initiate and sustain occupations they need to and want to pursue, when, where, how, and with whom. The broad concept of occupational participation includes occupational performance and occupational engagement. To understand what is meaningful and important for people's occupational participation, occupational therapists need to understand the historical factors that contribute to people's experiences (those of both individuals and collectives) and their relationships. They also need to understand that people's occupational possibilities are shaped by the broader context. Occupational therapists are guided to consider context at three levels: the micro, meso, and macro levels.

Collaborative Relationship-Focused Occupational Therapy: Major Concepts and Definitions

The second type of theoretical guideline presented in *Promoting Occupational Participation* is an approach called Collaborative Relationship-Focused Occupational Therapy. While the Canadian guidelines have maintained a central and enduring concern for client centeredness in occupational therapy, this approach represents a broadening of that focus to the *relationships* developed with people and collectives. The justification provided for adopting this broader concern for relationships is discussed in terms of the critiques of client centeredness, which can be categorized in three ways. First, when associated with a neoliberal perspective, the term *client* denotes commodification of the service user in terms of financial outcomes and individualism. Second, because the term *client* focuses on the service user, the characteristics of therapists and their contributions to the relationship can be overlooked. Specifically, their positionality and experiences of privilege or oppression and their emotional reactions to service users are often not attended to in the relationship. And third, drawing attention to client -centeredness can result in insufficient awareness being directed to the relational context. The relational context can include diversity in the relationships forged between individuals and collectives and their physical, social, cultural, historical, ancestral, and financial environments. It also includes "the interpersonal and systemic biases and discrimination that oppress individuals and communities according to factors, including race, ethnicity, dis/ability, being an immigrant or refugee, socioeconomic status, sex, gender, sexual orientation, and age, and how occupational therapists may be complicit in such discrimination" (Restall and Egan 2022, p. 100). By understanding the relationship context in this way, the Collaborative Relationship-Focused Occupational Therapy approach emphasizes human rights, justice, and equity and the structural and interpersonal factors that can shape them. As Restall and Egan explained, this approach "has greater potential to build and sustain relationships in which people feel safer, and that promote rights-based self-determination of individuals and collectives. Concerns regarding justice, equality, and rights, provide an essential background" (p. 99). The approach centers on relationships in which occupational therapists aim to work collaboratively with individuals and collectives to identify goals and priorities that are meaningful and important to them.

The approach is presented in *Promoting Occupational Participation* a flower-like diagram with collaborative relationship-focused occupational therapy in the center and four petal-like shapes surrounding it, each containing a key relational characteristic of the approach. The first key relational characteristic is *contextually relevant relationships*. This key characteristic emphasizes that the relationships developed between occupational therapists and the people they work with need to be founded on mutual respect and an appreciation that worldviews, values, and beliefs are varied among people. It warns against occupational therapists imposing, whether intentionally or unintentionally, their own perspectives and values, rather than listening with humility to those of the people they are working with. Critical self-awareness on the part of occupational therapists is essential. This includes awareness of their own personal beliefs and values, as well as of their social positionality, which creates often-unrecognized privileges or oppressions that are imposed by social beliefs and structures. Restall and Egan (2022) explained that the Global North outlook adopted by many countries, and which has been very influential in shaping occupational therapy's perspective, is founded on the principles of individualism, managerialism, and neoliberalism. Occupational therapists need to be aware of how the sociocultural context shapes their own perspectives and creates biases that, often without conscious awareness, can lead to therapist actions that are detrimental to people who are already structurally disadvantaged.

To be able to develop contextually relevant relationships, it is imperative that occupational therapists understand their own biases and stereotypical assumptions. As Restall and Egan (2022) contended, occupational therapists "have an obligation to disrupt both interpersonal and systemic oppression" (p. 103), and they promoted cultural humility as an important attitude to adopt. They defined cultural humility as comprising "life-long critical reflexivity by healthcare providers regarding social positioning, bias, and structural sources of privilege and oppression" (p. 103). Through cultural humility, occupational therapists can become aware of their own implicit and explicit biases and can value and respect the diverse worldviews, perspectives, values and beliefs, and ways of living of others.

In addition, occupational therapists also need to recognize that the structures in which they work influence what they do and are historically shaped. Referring to the Canadian context (and drawing parallels with other countries with similar worldviews and histories), Restall and Egan (2022) discussed the pervasiveness of White and Global North perspectives in the systems within which occupational therapists work. As they stated, "the influence of this epistemological dominance, combined with a prevailing history of exclusion, discounting, and structurally violent efforts to erase other ways of doing and being – such as has been experienced by Indigenous people in Canada – has been profound" (p. 103). They went on to explain that this influence has largely been invisible because it has been subsumed within ways of knowing, being, and doing that have been privileged, and that the outcomes of these discriminatory processes have become normalized and accepted. Consequently, they emphasized the need for occupational therapists to critically reflect on practices and the assumptions underpinning them, and on how the policies and procedures of organizations and institutions shape practice in terms of what is expected, allowed, promoted, and discouraged. Occupational therapists need to be aware of how these policies and expectations influence relationship building, particularly when those policies conflict with the client's expected cultural practices (e.g., gift giving). As they stated, occupational therapists "must recognize and address the forces that facilitate or constrain relationship building. This requires therapists to examine how stigmas, ableism, racism, and additional forms of oppression are enacted in systematic, intrapersonal, epistemic, and interpersonal practices and structures. It requires therapists' active engagement in addressing inequalities and injustices in everyday practice by changing policies and practices. Political and public advocacy and resistance to oppressions are essential" (p. 104).

The second key relational characteristic is *nuanced relationships*. Therapeutic relationships need to be contextually nuanced. This refers to the need for occupational therapists to be able to respond to the needs of the people they are working with from those people's own perspectives. When working with individuals, occupational therapists need to understand what is important to people and what their priorities are. They need to ensure that they do not just impose their own therapy priorities on the relationship. Therapeutic relationships also need to be temporally nuanced. Relationships take time to build. Depending upon the context, occupational therapists might have a long period of time to build relationships, or they might have to build them quickly over a short time. Restall and Egan (2022) reported that the institutional demands on occupational therapists' time often leave them less time to work with the people receiving services, which creates a dilemma for therapists about how best to use their time. However, the authors emphasized that being present and that deep and careful listening are important strategies for developing relationships when time is limited. Once developed, relationships also change over time and occupational therapists need to adapt with nuance to these changes. For example, in a rehabilitation context, goals will change over time as people's recovery progresses, and consequently, occupational therapists' roles will change.

The third key relational characteristic is *strives for safety in therapeutic relationships*. Occupational therapists need to ensure that they create therapeutic relationships in which the people they are working with feel safe. This includes physical, emotional, spiritual, and cultural safety. Occupational therapists need to minimize risk and prevent physical harm, which can occur either intentionally or unintentionally and can result from actions and omissions that cause harm through "ineffective, inappropriate, or missed opportunities for intervention" (Restall and Egan 2022, p. 105). Emotional safety requires trust and respect for people's cultural and spiritual beliefs and practices. Occupational therapists need to listen deeply to the concerns of individuals and collectives and be aware of the impact of structural discrimination and disadvantage on their survival strategies, relationships, and valued occupations. They also need to be aware of their own positions of power and privilege in therapeutic relationships and to take a humble and respectful approach to understanding the cultural practices, spiritual beliefs, and lives of the people with whom they work. In Canada the notion of cultural safety stems from discourse on the effects of the Western colonial healthcare system on Canadian Indigenous peoples. It acknowledges that the social, political, and historical contexts of healthcare have often not promoted health practices that are culturally safe. As Restall and Egan (2022) emphasized, "anti-racist, anti-oppressive, and trauma-informed approaches that recognize root causes of historical, intergenerational, and contemporary trauma are important. Culturally safer care involves therapists' consideration, analysis, and reduction of systemic power imbalances, discrimination, and colonisation. Occupational therapists have a duty to address these systemic issues that create barriers to safe occupational therapy practices" (p. 105).

To create safety in therapeutic relationships, occupational therapists must be trauma informed. Occupational therapists need to understand that trauma can be experienced by individuals, families, communities, and populations, and can be passed down through generations (referred to as *transgenerational* and *intergenerational* trauma). As Restall and Egan (2022) explained, "sources of trauma are diverse and can include violence in the form of power or threat against an individual or group, personal loss, war, or natural disaster" (p. 106). Violence can be interpersonal and structural, the latter being indirect and enshrined in social structures and resulting in unequal power and inequalities in life chances. Structural violence can manifest in the unequal distribution of and access to resources, inequalities in death and disability rates, and violation of human rights. Occupational therapists need to be careful that they do not perpetuate trauma through unsafe actions such as violations of relationship boundaries (which occurs when the relationship is organized to meet a therapist's own needs rather than those of the people using the service). Instead they need to create relationships of respectful, reciprocal, and culturally appropriate understanding.

The fourth key relational characteristic is *promotes rights-based self-determination*. Restall and Egan (2022) stated that a collaborative relationship that does this is one that "acknowledges people's entitlement to make decisions that affect their lives and their communities"

(p. 107). Occupational therapists need to underpin their therapeutic relationships with an absolute commitment to respecting the rights of individuals and collectives to self-determination. This involves acknowledging their capacities and strengths; listening to, acknowledging, and understanding their worldviews, values, and priorities; and engaging them in a shared decision-making process that provides information required for making informed choices. This last point might involve considering their health literacy and the social, political, cultural, economic, and environmental factors that can enable or restrict their choices.

Consistent with previous Canadian guidelines, Collaborative Relationship-Focused Occupational Therapy enshrines two enduring values: (1) it places the people occupational therapists work with at the center of the approach; and (2) throughout the discussions of the approach, occupational therapy's aspirations of achieving equity and justice are embedded. To address this second value, occupational therapists are implored to attend to the structural barriers presented by the social, economic, and political organization of society that create inequity and impede justice. Factors that can challenge occupational therapists when enacting the collaborative relationship-focused occupational therapy approach are the predominance of the biomedical approach and its associated Western-based social norms, a paucity of time, and the need for structural competency. First, regarding the biomedical approach, this perspective influences the way many services are organized and shapes their priorities, goals, and expectations. A biomedical perspective can also be internalized by occupational therapists because it forms the dominant health perspective of many societies, and this can limit the possibilities that occupational therapists might consider. In terms of time, the demands and expectations of practice settings can limit the time available for relationship building and collaboratively identifying meaningful goals and priorities. Finally, social and structural factors can limit the capacity of individuals and collectives to achieve their goals and priorities and can limit their occupational participation. Second, for occupational therapists to promote equity and justice, they need to develop structural competency. Restall and Egan (2022) identified four components of structural competency: (1) developing an awareness of how society's structures contribute to the health, behaviors, choices, and occupational possibilities of people; (2) understanding how occupational therapists' clinical actions and decisions are shaped by their social positions and other economic and sociopolitical forces; (3) remembering that the societal structures that create and reinforce inequities should not be conflated with the notion of culture; and (4) using interventions such as advocacy to address structural violence.

Collaborative relationships in occupational therapy require self-knowledge on the part of therapists as well as the ability to understand and respect the diversity of worldviews, values, and beliefs of the individuals and collectives they are working with. To create the conditions in which collaborative relationships can flourish, occupational therapists need to listen with humility to people's stories and "earn the privilege of hearing people's histories, present-day realities, and future aspirations" (Restall and Egan 2022, p. 109). They also need to work at the institutional level, advocating for services that allow the time and resources needed to provide enabling and relevant occupational therapy and for systems that facilitate equality and justice.

At an educational level, graduates need to undertake critical reflection on their own worldviews, values, and beliefs, as well as on the perspectives and practices of occupational therapy. They need to understand the structural factors in society that promote and constrain occupational participation, equality, and justice, as well as the effects of colonization on the health and well-being of marginalized groups and the effects of issues such as "racism, ableism, sexism, heteronormativism, ageism, and additional sources of domination emanating from structural violence that often goes unrecognized" (Restall and Egan 2022, p. 109). They need to develop the moral courage to disrupt existing structures that limit participation and to advocate for structures that promote equality and justice.

Canadian Occupational Therapy Interrelational Practice Process Framework: Major Concepts and Definitions

The third guideline presented in *Promoting Occupational Participation* is the Canadian Occupational Therapy Inter-Relational Practice Process (COTIPP) Framework. In its development, the COTIPP built on previous Canadian practice frameworks, drew upon diverse perspectives and experiences, and considered ways to orient practice toward justice and equity. It aims to outline an occupational therapy practice that is collaborative, interrelational, and rights based. Such a practice requires respectful partnerships and recognition of the multiple relationships among diverse entities, including "all beings, ancestors, the natural environment, inanimate objects, knowledge, ideas, beliefs, customs, protocols, and identities" (Restall et al. 2022, p. 121). It recognizes international and national human rights conventions and declarations, particularly those advocating for vulnerable groups such as children, Indigenous peoples, and people with disabilities. It promotes rights-based self-determination of individuals and collectives, attending to societal structures that constrain choice and occupational possibilities and endeavoring to promote justice and occupational participation.

At the centre of the COTIPP is the *essential underlying process* to build and sustain relationships. In working toward this essential process, three *foundational processes* are outlined: seek understanding about context; reflect, critically reflect, and reason; and use justice-, equity-, and rights-based lenses. Six *action domains* are undertaken: (1) connect; (2) seek understanding and define purpose; (3) explore occupational participation; (4) co-design priorities, goals, outcomes, and plans; (5) trial the plan, explore change, and refine the plan; and (6) plan for transition. In discussing the various components of the model, Restall et al. (2022) explained that they are mutually influencing and "flow into and across each other" (p. 123). Three assumptions about occupational therapy underpin the COTIPP framework: (1) it is different in every context; (2) it often (but not always) has a defined beginning and end; and (3) it is most often an iterative process that is responsive to context and relationships (but can follow a step-by-step process if that is most appropriate).

At the center of the framework is the essential, underlying practice of building and sustaining relationships with individuals and collectives. This is done through collaborative, relationship-focused practice, which requires occupational therapists to practice with respect and trust, promote choice and collaboration, and attend to (and attempt to minimize) structures that create power imbalances.

The first of the three foundational processes is *seek understanding about context*. The COTIPP conceptualizes the various aspects of the contexts in which people live and participate as mutually influencing. The notion of context is understood broadly and includes "history, geographic location, the natural and built environment, social and economic laws, legislation and policies, organizational policies and rules, social and cultural norms and expectations, social identities, secular and religious beliefs, prevailing societal attitudes and behaviors, networks, and power relations within and among collectives (families, groups, communities, and populations)" (Restall et al. 2022, p. 124).

The COTIPP specifically attends to three aspects of context: the therapist context, the practice context, and the individual's and collective's context. The therapist context is presented first. Occupational therapists need to attend to their own context (self-context), which includes their social identities, histories, and experiences, and the unearned privileges and oppressions associated with these. They need to consider how various aspects of their identities might contribute to their relationships with others. Aspects of their identities to consider include race; ethnicity; sexual identity, orientation, and expression; dis/ability; social class; religion; and history. Through critical reflexivity, they try to uncover their own conscious and unconscious biases and then use an increased understanding of these biases to reduce their own potential for perpetuation of systemic injustices and inequalities. They attend to the degree to which their own personal and professional perspectives have been shaped by the internalization of beliefs stemming from macro-level structures such as colonialism, racism, ableism, and sexism, to name a few. They need to be alert to the potential to cause harm through perpetuation of power imbalances associated with such macro-level structures. They need to adopt a stance of "ongoing humble self-reflection and intellectual humility" (Restall et al. 2022, p. 125), through which they aim to increase awareness of their own taken-for-granted perspectives and beliefs and the potential influence of these on the people with whom they work.

Next, occupational therapists must endeavor to understand the practice context—how it is organized and the degree to which it may constrict the practice of occupational therapy and influence occupational possibilities. They need to be aware of how Global North attitudes support the organization and structures of practice environments and how the history of colonization, racism, and oppression contributes to structural inequality and the power imbalance inherent in services. They need to use the socioecological and social determinants of health and well-being perspectives to critique how their services are organized and delivered. Occupational therapists also need to understand occupational therapy's colonial roots and its complicity with colonial, racist, and oppressive systems, and the need to disrupt "existing systems and epistemologies with actions that further justice, equity, and rights" (Restall et al. 2022, p. 125). By understanding the various internal and external factors influencing the practice context, occupational therapists can work with others to address and minimize barriers to equitable services and facilitate access to resources. They need to be able to align with the perspectives of the communities with which they are working.

The final aspect of context considered within building and sustaining relationships is the context of the individuals and collectives accessing occupational therapy services. While attempting to understand these contexts, occupational therapists recognize that they can never be fully known. While acknowledging that their understanding will only be partial, occupational therapists adopt an approach in which they are continuously curious about and attentive to changes that occur throughout the process of therapy. Occupational therapists need to consider that all three aspects of context—their own, that of the practice context, and those of the people accessing services—will always have aspects that remain hidden to them, whether through taken-for-granted assumptions, convention, or contexts that are foreign to them. Through an attitude of humble curiosity, they can remain open to building and sustaining relationships based on mutual respect and understanding.

The second foundational process for building and sustaining relationships is *reflect, critically reflect, and reason*. Restall et al. (2022) used the work of Donald Schön (1983) to discuss reflective practice. Schön coined the term *reflection in action* to refer to the capacity of professionals to consciously reflect on what they are doing while they are doing it. Restall et al. explained that this allows occupational therapists to observe what is working well and what is not and to make adjustments there and then to improve the process of therapy. Schön also used the term *reflection-on-action* for reflecting after the action has taken place. Restall et al. emphasized that, when reflecting on their action, occupational therapists need to apply their reflection to both specific sessions and their practice in general. As they stated, "therapists must understand their own social positions, histories, culture, values, and beliefs and be aware of how these factors affect both reflection and practice" (p. 128). They recommended that reflection after action can be enhanced by undertaking it with trusted colleagues and mentors.

Restall et al. (2022) then explained that critical reflection differs from reflection by being based on critical theory. Critical reflection is directed to the systems in which occupational therapy is provided as well as to the broader society, and it specifically attends to issues of power and equity. Some examples of issues that might surface through critical reflection are organizational policies that limit alternatives to in-person services and standard hours of service provision, and racist or ableist social attitudes that limit people's access to work and public services such as transport. Such insights can then form the basis for actions such as advocacy to address such issues and reduce barriers. The term *occupational consciousness* (Ramugondo 2015) refers to the everyday actions people use to resist and challenge dominant practices that sustain unequal power relations. Occupational therapists can use this concept to help them consider the degree to which their own actions perpetuate or resist systems of oppression. An example is consideration of the appropriateness of standardized assessments (generated from Global North perspectives) for people whose worldviews have different perspectives on occupation, health and well-being, and human development. Restall et al. proposed the general question, "how can every day occupations become acts of resistance by identifying new ways of collaboratively exploring occupations from varied perspectives?" (p. 131.) They contended that action can be employed to transform injustices when using a "decolonial lens and socio-political practice" (p. 131).

When discussing reason, Restall et al. (2022) placed a spotlight on practice reasoning, which they defined as "occupational therapists' thinking and decision-making processes that guide quality and ethical practice" (p. 131), and they highlighted that this definition emphasizes the central role of ethical decision-making in practice. Because of the complexity and context dependence of practice reasoning, Restall et al. stressed again the importance of occupational therapists reflecting on and becoming aware of their own taken-for-granted assumptions and worldviews for improving it. Occupational therapists also need to listen carefully to the perspectives, beliefs, and desires of the people with whom they work when making practice decisions. They need to reflect critically on the practice settings within which they work and consider the degree to which those settings facilitate or constrain the best possible and most ethical outcomes for the people they work with.

The third foundational process for building and sustaining relationships is *rse justice-, equity-, and rights-based lenses*. Embedded in the COTIPP is the imperative for occupational therapists to uphold the rights of people to justice and equal access to occupational participation. Occupational therapists have the obligation and moral and ethical responsibility to promote equity and justice and preserve the rights of the people with whom they work. They need to look for situations and social structures that can constrain people's rights, access to justice, and equitable occupational participation. They need to work at the macro level as well as the micro level. The concept of occupational justice (Townsend and Whiteford 2000) applies an occupational lens to social justice issues, and the World Federation of Occupational Therapists (WFOT) makes it clear that occupational therapists have an obligation to promote occupational justice because occupational rights are a manifestation of human rights. In adopting justice-, equity-, and rights-based lenses, occupational therapists will be alert to instances and situations that erode occupational justice and people's right to occupational participation.

Finally, the *six action domains* of the COTIPP are: (1) connect; (2) seek understanding and define purpose; (3) explore occupational participation; (4) co-design priorities, goals, outcomes, and plans; (5) trial the plan, explore change, and refine the plan; and (6) plan for transition. Restall et al. (2022) emphasized that, while each action domain is described separately, they are interrelated and are best conceptualized as comprising a fluid process (rather than being sequential steps). An occupational therapist may be engaged in multiple action domains at one time. For example, when exploring occupational participation, occupational therapists are most likely to also develop an understanding of the individual's or collective's priorities and desires as well as building a connection with them. The authors also clarified that not all six action domains will be appropriate in every situation. For example, the people occupational therapists are working with might largely be looking to clarify their priorities and goals and not wish to trial a plan. Also, where involvement is ongoing, planning for transition will not be required. The context in which the encounter occurs will also determine how much time is spent with people. Consequently, some situations might mean occupational therapists undertake many of the action domains in a short period of time, and in other situations they could be working on various action domains multiple times over months or years.

The first action domain identified is *connect*. This refers to occupational therapists' first meeting with individuals and collectives, signaling the beginning of a trusting, collaborative relationship. Regardless of how this is instigated (e.g., referral), occupational therapists are responsible for promoting equal access for a diversity of people to be able to commence occupational therapy. Being able to connect with people may be impeded by current and past trauma and previous negative experiences with government and health and social services. During the connect phase, occupational therapists need to consider their competencies, experiences, and conflicts of interest and clarify what occupational therapy can offer, as well as establishing informed and noncoercive consent. The decision to proceed with occupational therapy must be a collaborative one.

The second action domain is *seek understanding and define purpose*. This action domain is characterized by deep listening to the individual's and collective's concerns, priorities, goals, beliefs, dreams, and aspirations regarding occupational participation. Occupational therapists seek to understand what individuals and collectives hope for and expect from therapy and to learn through narrative about their histories and experiences.

The third action domain is *explore occupational participation*. The conditions for exploring occupational participation are co-created by therapists and the individuals and collectives with whom they are working. Together they determine how those people's current occupational concerns, aspirations, and possibilities will be approached. For example, they might cooperatively deem formal or informal assessments or different types of evaluations most appropriate. These might include "interviews, questionnaires, observations in people's environments, formal assessment tools, sharing circles, and community forums" (Restall et al. 2022, p. 136). Using collaborative approaches and deep listening is important for understanding occupational participation needs and possible solutions from multiple perspectives. These different perspectives might be gained from family members and care partners as well as from members of interprofessional and interdisciplinary teams. Additional perspectives can be gained from people working in other areas, such as education, social service, and justice. This approach to gaining multiple perspectives always needs to consider privacy, confidentiality, and cultural norms.

The fourth action domain is *co-design priorities, goals, outcomes, and plans*. Co-design is a central principle of the COTIPP. Rather than making decisions about what they think is best, occupational therapists need to understand the concerns and aspirations of the people they are working with regarding occupational participation. They need to work with them to understand their priorities for occupational participation and to jointly identify meaningful goals and outcomes. Restall et al. (2022) proposed that priorities and action plans are more likely to be appropriate than goal setting when working with communities. When making action plans, occupational therapists need to consider that these could be targeted at the individual, collective, or system level.

The fifth action domain is *trial the plan, explore change, and refine the plan*. This action domain is about bringing the plan to life. It involves trialing the action that has been planned and "co-monitoring" it with the individual or collective to determine its effect on occupational participation. The course of action is co-monitored in terms of people's perceptions of progress and experiences of safety. Adjustments and refinements are made as needed, to both the plan and the priorities, goals, and outcomes underpinning it. Where organizational policies and circumstances limit the time available for occupational therapy, therapists need to be clear with the individuals and collectives about how these constraints will impact the time and resources available. Therapists also need to advocate for change in structures and any other factors at the micro, meso, and macro levels that could restrict equitable access to and utilization of occupational therapy.

The sixth and final action domain is *plan for transition*. This pertains to transitioning from occupational therapy services. This process of closure entails reflecting on and articulating what

TABLE 7.1 ■ **Components of the Canadian Occupational Therapy Inter-Relational Practice Process (COTIPP)**

Essential underlying process	Build and sustain relationships
Foundational processes	Seek understanding about context • Therapist context • Practice context • Individual's/collective's context Reflect, critically reflect, and reason Use justice-, equity-, and rights-based lenses
Action domains	Connect Seek understanding and define purpose Explore occupational participation Co-design priorities, goals, outcomes, and plans Trial the plan, explore change, and refine the plan Plan for transition

has been achieved together and determining the next steps for the individuals or collectives. This might include referrals to other services or recommendations pertaining to actions to build on and sustain gains made. For people experiencing deteriorating health conditions, this may include strategies for maintaining occupational participation as capacities and circumstances change.

In summary, the COTIPP framework aims to guide occupational therapists to create an occupational therapy practice that is collaborative, interrelational, and rights based (see Table 7.1). It centers on building and sustaining relationships that are based on a deep understanding of the broader historical and sociopolitical context in which occupational therapy occurs. Occupational therapists need to be aware of their own positionalities, organizational policies and practices, and contexts and experiences of the people with whom they work that create injustices that impede occupational participation, and work to address them. They work collaboratively with people to achieve the outcomes they need and desire in their lives.

Overall, taken together, the CanMOP, the collaborative relationship-focused practice approach, and the COTIPP framework form the current suite of guidelines published by the CAOT. They aim to provide guidance to Canadian occupational therapists working in a contemporary society that has come to recognize the historical roots of continuing injustices, oppressions, and inequities entrenched in its sociopolitical landscape born of colonialism. This demands a social justice approach from occupational therapists in everyday practice to work to address the social, systemic, and structural drivers of inequities. A critical lens emphasizes the intersectionality of a range of factors including gender, disability, sexuality, ethnicity, and socioeconomic status that are associated with sustained inequities in health, well-being, and occupational participation. Occupational therapists are guided to listen deeply to their clients and respond at the micro, meso, and macro levels of context to promote equity, justice, and rights-based occupational participation. A case illustration is provided in Box 7.2 of Christina, an occupational therapist working with Andrea to facilitate her occupational participation in her community.

Historical Description of the Canadian Guidelines' Development

The CanMOP is the latest model in a long line of official guidelines published by the CAOT. Egan and Restall (2022) explained that the first national Canadian model was published in the

BOX 7.2 ■ Case Illustration

Christina is an occupational therapist who has worked for 15 years in an outpatient rehabilitation center for people with spinal cord injuries. She recently received a referral for Andrea, a 13-year-old girl who was diagnosed with paraplegia after a car accident when she was 2 years old. The referral requested that occupational therapy conduct a home visit to investigate why Andrea is not attending school. Christina has worked with Andrea before and knows she comes from a low socioeconomic background and lives with her mother and two siblings in a hilly area. The rehabilitation team has noticed for a long time that Andrea often has poor hygiene when she attends rehabilitation sessions, and she often misses sessions because of difficulties traveling to the center.

When Christina came to Andrea's house, she found that it was located above the road on sloping ground and was separated from the road by a gully. It did not have any adaptations to improve access. Andrea's mother carries her in her arms from the road, across the gully, and up to the house. She has difficulty doing this because Andrea is too heavy for her. She also needs someone else from the family to carry the wheelchair. Inside the house, the bathroom is not well equipped, and they do not have access to hot water. Andrea's grandmother, two aunts, and their families, who support her in her everyday occupations, live in the house next door. There is a stop for the school bus down the road, but she cannot use the bus because it is not accessible.

When Christina submitted her assessment report to the rehabilitation team, they suggested that the ideal scenario would be to apply for subsidized government housing for people with disabilities so that Andrea and her mother could have an accessible house in an area with appropriate public transport. However, looking through the lens of the CanMOP, Christina was uncomfortable with this proposal and knew that some information was missing. Guided by the COTIPP, in a second visit to the home she purposefully tried to deeply connect and understand the priorities of Andrea and her family. Christina found out that Andrea's mother and siblings did not want to move from their house, because they had always lived near their family and felt safe in that environment. Christina also came to understand the issue of poor hygiene. Andrea indicated that attending to school was very valuable for her, and it was the only place she had friends. However, her mother explained that, because it was so difficult for Andrea to wash herself at home and she was so ashamed of her poor hygiene, she had become reluctant to attend school. Considering what was meaningful for Andrea and her family, Christina worked with them to collaboratively identify goals for occupational therapy. At the micro level, Christina organized to modify the environment by having a ramp built across the gully from the road to their house and adapting the bathroom so that Andrea could access it more easily. At the meso level, Christina advocated with the local authorities to provide access to hot water and negotiated with the school to assist Andrea with adapted transport to facilitate her attendance to school. At the macro level, Christina advocated for a scheme for funding community connection events in Andrea and her extended family's community so that the community could strengthen its cohesion. For example, this might enable it to have community art events in which the schoolchildren could play a central role. She also advocated for a change in housing policy that would honor people's connection with their communities.

Occupational Therapy Guidelines for Client-Centred Practice (Department of National Health and Welfare and Canadian Association of Occupational Therapists 1983). These guidelines were based on the occupational performance models that were common at the time (see Chapter 3) and centered on the notion of occupational performance (which was also referred to as *function*). These models categorized occupational performance into the performance areas of self-care, productivity, and leisure.

The next major development in the CAOT guidelines was the publication of *Enabling Occupation: An Occupational Therapy Perspective* (CAOT 1997), and the model presented in that text became known as the Canadian Model of Occupational Performance (CMOP). The CMOP continued the categorizetion of occupational performance into the areas of self-care, productivity, and leisure. These areas of occupational performance were considered the outcome of the interaction between the characteristics of a person (presented as physical, affective, and cognitive performance components, with a spiritual core) and the environment (conceptualized as having physical, social, cultural, and institutional aspects).

In 2007, *Enabling Occupation II* was published, and the CMOP was developed into the Canadian Model of Occupational Performance and Engagement (CMOP-E), expanding its concern beyond occupational performance to incorporate the concept of engagement, noting that people could be engaged in occupation without performing it. As illustration, the authors gave the example of a father and his disabled son doing triathlons together. While the father performed the components of the triathlon, the son participated in (was engaged in) the activities by being towed in a boat or being pulled behind the bike when cycling and his father when running. The concept of engagement was broken down into its "nature (active or passive), intensity (sporadic or constant), degree of establishment (novel or long-standing and established), extent (fully engaged or barely attentive), competency of performance (novice or expert), and so on" (Townsend and Polatajko 2007, p. 25).

The theme running through all these Canadian models since 1983 is client centeredness. As Restall and Egan (2022) explained, "Canadian occupational therapists were among the first health professionals to embrace client-centred practice as a key approach to their work" (p. 99). However, given that Western/Global North notions of occupational therapy focus on the individual, it is unsurprising that the diagrammatic representations of these earlier client-centered models centered on the individual person. One of the major changes that occurred between the CMOP and the CMOP-E relates to the definition of the client. This reflects the changing nature of occupational therapists' practice and the increasing diversity of occupational therapists' roles, as well as the broader society's changing concepts relating to health. While maintaining the original diagram with the person in the center, the CMOP-E emphasized that the *client* was not just an individual, but could be individuals, families, groups, communities, organizations (including agencies, clubs and associations, and other government, corporate, or nongovernment organizations) and populations. Consequently, occupational therapy intervention could be aimed at any of these levels. Client centeredness and a broad understanding of the term *client* remain embedded in the CanMOP through constant use of the phrase *individuals and collectives* and the specific listing of the six types of clients.

The evolution from a focus on client centeredness to one on relationships is also evident in discussion of Collaborative Relationship-Focused Occupational Therapy. Key features of client centeredness contribute to the contemporary concept of collaborative, relationship-focused practice in occupational therapy: a holistic view of people as active participants who are empowered to make informed choices, the importance of working collaboratively with people, and respecting people's right to make choices about their own needs and occupational therapy services. Added to these are an emphasis on fostering trust, attention to power structures that pervade both therapist–client relationships and sociopolitical systems, and the importance of promoting human rights, justice, and equality.

Regarding the CanMOP, Egan and Restall (2022) presented six essential enhancements that had been incorporated since the earlier models: "a) an explicit focus on occupational participation, b) removal of categorization, c) explicit consideration of meaning, d) advanced consideration of performance components and the environment, e) explicit consideration of history, and f) explicit consideration of occupational possibilities" (p. 88).

First, the CanMOP focuses explicitly on occupational participation by placing it at the center of the model. By making this broader notion of occupational participation explicit, the model aims to ensure that adequate consideration is given to the meaning and context of occupations. While occupational performance might center an occupational therapist's attention on performance in the service context, the concept of occupational performance refocuses attention on the contexts in which people live. As Egan and Restall (2022) stated, "[occupational therapists] also attend to whether the person can do the occupation with the people they wish, within the environment that is important to them, and can continue to do so following discontinuation of service" (p. 88).

Second, the CanMOP does not categorize occupation into the performance areas that were characteristic of the earlier Canadian models. These areas largely reflect assumptions from the Global North about the purpose of occupations, and using them meant other important occupations that did not fit neatly into these categories, such as transportation, navigating social services, and volunteering in the community, might frequently be overlooked.

While categorization relates to the purpose of occupations, the third essential enhancement pertains to the meaning of occupation. Consideration of meaning is critical to the perspective and practice of occupational therapy. The CanMOP guides occupational therapists to make it a central aspect of their reasoning. Egan and Restall (2022) linked the meaning of occupation to spirituality and implored occupational therapists to be receptive to the spiritual as it is core to a person's sense of meaning and purpose.

The fourth essential enhancement is advanced consideration of performance components and the environment. While the earlier Canadian models made explicit the physical, cognitive, and affective performance components, the CanMOP assumes that occupational therapists have an expert understanding of these performance components, but it does not specifically include them in the model. The CanMOP also highlights the need to understand how characteristics of the environment affect the occupational performance of specific individuals and collectives. It emphasizes how the micro, meso, and macro levels of the environment impact one another and influence the possibilities for occupational performance.

The fifth essential enhancement is explicit consideration of history. It attends to an individual's history using the principles of the Life Course perspective in which the timing of events in a person's life and their interconnectedness with others is emphasized. It considers the history of collectives such as communities, considering how past events impact the present.

The sixth essential enhancement is explicit consideration of occupational possibilities. The CanMOP is the first Canadian model that includes the concept of occupational possibilities. By highlighting the layers of context at the micro, meso, and macro levels, the CanMOP guides occupational therapists to consider the realities of what is available to individuals and collectives.

Another way the CanMOP differs from earlier Canadian guidelines is through its explicit focus on the Indigenous peoples of Canada and the history and ongoing legacy of colonization. It emphasizes that occupational therapy needs to be aware of and recognize its context within a colonial nation. Acknowledgment of the current effects on people of the colonial past is central to the five principles that underpin *Promoting Occupational Participation*:

1. Recognize the unique position of Indigenous peoples in Canada, the history and ongoing legacy of colonization, and the context of occupational therapy in a colonial nation
   This principle emphasizes the need for occupational therapists to promote the principles of human rights and justice for Indigenous peoples and to recognize structural injustice.
2. Be inclusive of, and relevant to, diverse people, communities, societies, and systems
   The most recent guidelines continue to emphasize that the people who receive services from occupational therapists can be individuals, families, groups, communities, and populations. However, in comparison with earlier guidelines, they provide more guidance for working with groups, communities, and populations.
3. Place a holistic perspective on occupation and occupational participation at the core of what occupational therapists do

Taking such a holistic perspective on occupation and occupational participation requires that occupational therapists recognize the complexity, particularly in relation to the social structures that produce and maintain inequities.

4. **Fairly represent a range of worldviews, cultural practices, and values, recognizing multiple sources of intersectionality**
   Occupational therapists need to be inclusive of a diversity of ways of thinking, perceiving, and being, and of values, worldviews, and cultural practices. They need to be aware of how such diversity can form the basis of inequities and how multiple differences can intersect to compound inequality.

5. **Take an affirmational, strengths-based, healing-centered, and trauma-informed approach**
   Occupational therapists need to practice in a way that recognizes, affirms, and encourages individuals and communities to build upon their strengths and abilities and to use their resources to enhance their well-being. They need to be aware of and acknowledge trauma, but also ensure that they do not perpetuate it in the way they practice. They need to remain strengths and wellness based in their practice.

Egan and Restall (2022) provide comparisons with models used in other sectors. In addition to the *International Classification of Functioning, Disability and Health (ICF)* and the Disability Creation Process (DCP), they identified three conceptual approaches with which the CanMOP is compatible:

- The Social Model of Disability was developed in response to the biomedical perspective, which equated disability with impairment. A biomedical notion of disability presents a normative view of body structures and functions and understands disability as resulting from abnormal body functions and structures. Instead, the Social Model of Disability argues that people are disabled by society's organization and structures. People face inequitable opportunities to participate in occupations because of factors such as social practices, social attitudes, the design of built environments and objects, and the organization of social institutions. The Social Model of Disability advocates for changes to social structures and practices rather than remediation of impairment, and the CanMOP aligns with this approach by advocating for analysis of micro, meso, and macro contextual elements and collaborative problem-solving "while working to dismantle systemic injustice" (p. 91).

- The Recovery Model was developed in mental health and "denotes the right of people with a diagnosis of mental illness to have a personally gratifying, dignified life with community connections and relationships regardless of diagnostic labels or impairments" (p. 92). The CanMOP aligns with this approach in that it focuses on people's right to live meaningful and purposeful lives, full of occupational possibilities, regardless of their capacities, diagnostic labels, and impairments.

- Critical theory perspectives refer to an array of different theories such as critical race theory, feminism, and queer theory. Critical theories identify and address the power imbalances in society that produce discrimination and oppression, "with the ultimate goal of dismantling these to produce societies where differences are recognized and embraced" (p. 92). Particularly highlighted is critical disability theory, which rejects the ablest notion that inequity of participation is due to body structures and functions. It particularly attends to the intersection of multiple identities that compound oppression, such as race, gender, sexuality, and age. The CanMOP is compatible with these critical theories in that it attends to multiple identities of people and collectives, it is based on the real experiences of people rather than abstract notions, and it aims to identify and disrupt aspects of the macro-level context that impede and block occupational participation.

Memory Aid

See Box 7.3.

BOX 7.3 ■ Memory Aid

Occupational Therapist Personal Reflection

In what ways do my identities lead to unearned privilege or oppression? (Consider factors such as the practice context, social position, ethnicity, gender, sexual orientation, age, education, income, history, religion, embodiment.)

How might my identities affect my relationships with people whose social identities are similar to or different from mine?

In what ways do my practice context and profession perpetuate and entrench racism, sexism, ableism, ageism, heteronormativism, classism, and other sources of oppression?

Using the CanMOP

Identify the occupations that the client (individual or collective) needs or wishes to pursue. What are the circumstances in which the client would do them? (How, when, where, and with whom)

What does each of those occupations mean to the client and what purpose does it serve in their lives? (Consider the needs for survival and safety, autonomy, relatedness, and competence.)

■ How do past, present, and hoped-for future relationships influence the purpose and meaning of those occupations? (Consider relationships between people; their physical environments, histories, ancestors, cultures, knowledges, social, political, and economic structures; and the natural world.)

■ For individuals, how do the histories of their lives (Life Course) influence the meaning and purpose of occupations to them?

■ For communities, how is the community's history influencing the meaning and purpose of occupations for them?

Collaboratively explore occupational possibilities in terms of accessing, initiating, and sustaining occupations.

■ Are there any unexamined assumptions about what certain types of people can do that need to be challenged? (For individuals, these include aspects of a person's physical, affective, and cognitive structures and functions, and their beliefs, values, spirituality, and social identities. For collectives, these include the family or community's resources and utilization of resources, shared histories, values, and beliefs as well as interrelationships.)

■ What changes need to be made to the micro, meso, and macro contexts to facilitate occupational participation?

   ■ Micro context—consider intergenerational and ancestral influences, family, friends, schoolmates, teachers, co-workers, health and social service providers, and community relationships.

   ■ Meso context—consider policies and procedures of system structures such as healthcare and social service organizations and their programs.

   ■ Macro context—consider social and cultural values and beliefs reinforced by broader socioeconomic and political governance structures.

■ What strategies could be used to work collectively to dismantle social structures that limit occupational possibilities?

Major Works

Egan M, Restall G, eds. Promoting Occupational Participation: Collaborative Relationship Focused Occupational Therapy. CAOT; 2022.

Summary

In this chapter we presented the model, approach, and framework provided in *Promoting Occupational Participation: Collaborative Relationship Focused Occupational Therapy*, outlining the current position of the Canadian Association of Occupational Therapy. Respectively, these are the CanMOP, Collaborative Relationship Focused-Occupational Therapy, and the COTIPP framework. Together they aim to guide occupational therapists to provide holistic services to individuals and collectives while also working at a structural level to create a more just and equitable society the fosters occupational participation and leads to greater well-being.

These guidelines build upon the previous models and frameworks that emphasized client centeredness and occupational performance and engagement. Building on this foundation of client centeredness, these latest guidelines emphasize relationships and the historical and contemporary factors that contribute to structural justice. By focusing on relationships, the current guidelines bring therapists into the spotlight as well as clients, prompting therapists to explore their own positionality as well as that of their clients. The guidelines also draw upon the work of the Truth and Reconciliation Commission of Canada in raising awareness of the current impact of the colonial past for First Nation, Métis, and Inuit peoples through systemic factors that reduce health and limit access to life-sustaining and meaningful occupations. Specifically, the guidelines emphasize the pervasiveness of Western/Global North worldviews, marked by individualism, objective scientific rationality, and human dominance over nature, on all aspects of certain societies and on the profession of occupational therapy. Working to embrace a broad range of worldviews is vital for promoting meaningful and purposeful occupational participation.

References

Bronfenbrenner U. Making Human Beings Human: Bioecological Perspectives on Human Development. Sage; 2004.

Department of National Health and Welfare, Canadian Association of Occupational Therapists. Guidelines for the client-Centred practice of Occupational Therapy. H39-33/ 1983E ed. Ottawa: Department of National Health and Welfare; 1983.

Egan M, Restall G. The Canadian model of occupational participation. In: Egan M, Restall G, eds. Promoting Occupational Participation: Collaborative Relationship Focused Occupational Therapy. CAOT; 2022:73–95.

Laliberte Rudman D. Occupational terminology: occupational possibilities. J Occup Sci. 2010;17(1):55–59. doi:10.1080/14427591.2010.9686673

Ramugondo EL. Occupational consciousness. J Occup Sci. 2015 Oct 2;22(4):488–501. doi:10.1080/14427591.2015.1042516

Restall G, Egan M. Collaborative relationship-focused occupational therapy. In: Egan M, Restall G, eds. Promoting Occupational Participation: Collaborative Relationship Focused Occupational Therapy. CAOT; 2022:97–117.

Restall G, Egan M, Valavaar, K, Phenix A, Slack C. Canadian Occupational Therapy Inter-relational Practice Process Framework. In: Egan M, Restall G, eds. Promoting Occupational Participation: Collaborative Relationship Focused Occupational Therapy. CAOT; 2022:119–150.

Schön D. The Reflective Practitioner: How Professionals Think in Action. Basic Books; 1983.

Townsend EA, Polatajko HJ. Advancing an Occupational Therapy Vision for Health, Well-Being, and Justice Through Occupation. CAOT; 2007.

Trentham B, Laliberte Rudman D, Smith H, Phenix A. The socio-political and historical context of occupational therapy in Canada. In: Egan M, Restall G, eds. Promoting Occupational Participation: Collaborative Relationship Focused Occupational Therapy. CAOT; 2022:31–55.

Willcock A, Townsend EA. Occupational terminology interactive dialogue. J Occup Sci. 2000;7(2):84–86. doi:10.1080/14427591.2000.9686470

World Health Organization. Social determinants of health. 2022. World Health Organization. https://www.who.int/health-topics/social-determinants-of-health#tab=tab_1

CHAPTER 8

Kawa Model

CHAPTER CONTENTS

Main Concepts and Definitions of Terms   157

Elements of the River   160

The River Metaphor   163

Historical Description of the Model's Development   165

Japanese Culture Context   165
  Centrality of the Individual   166
  Occupational Beings   166
  Reconceptualizing Occupation   167

Development of the Model   168

Use of the Model in Practice   170

Memory Aid   171

Major Works   172

Conclusion   172

References   172

The Kawa (River in Japanese) model was developed by Michael Iwama, a Japanese-Canadian occupational therapist and social scientist, in conjunction with a group of Japanese occupational therapists. The Kawa model was presented at various conferences in the early 2000s and the main text outlining the model was published in 2006. Therefore it is one of the more recently developed models in this book (excluding more recent versions of previously developed models). The model was originally developed in response to a perceived need for an occupational therapy model that was appropriate to and useful in Japanese occupational therapy practice contexts. Therefore the challenge for Western readers when learning about this model is to understand it in the context of the culture within and for which it was developed. The Kawa model uses the metaphor of a river with various elements such as water, rock, driftwood, and the river floor and river walls. The potential trap for many readers is to take this metaphor and its elements and view them from an individualist perspective. Understood in this way, the model could look like any other occupational therapy model that deals with the person, environment, and occupation. However, by understanding the assumptions about the nature of self and agency that are embedded within collectivist cultures, such as Japanese and various Indigenous societies, Western readers are better able to understand the significance of the various elements of this model. To facilitate this process, we make comments throughout the description of the model that emphasize a culturally appropriate understanding of each phenomenon. Reference is also made to the distinction Iwama made between *collectivist* and *existential* perspectives. The former is the perspective characterized by many East Asian and indigenous cultures. The latter characterizes the individualist approach common in Western cultures.

Main Concepts and Definitions of Terms

The Kawa model is structured around the metaphor of a river and its elements. It uses the image of the water flowing through a river to represent "life energy" or "life flow." In this model the purpose of occupational therapy is to facilitate this life flow in the context of a harmonious balance with all aspects of the river. The river itself is used to describe a person's life history (Fig. 8.1), and cross sections of the river at different times in the person's history (Figs. 8.2 and 8.3) can reveal the elements in the river. These elements are the river floor and walls, rocks, driftwood, and the spaces between these. Each element represents an aspect of the person's life circumstances. The water flows through the channels created by the relative positions and sizes of the other elements. Change can occur in the river by alteration of the position, size, and shape of the elements to increase or decrease the flow of the water, representing a change in life flow. This potential for change is the basis for occupational therapy intervention.

The river is used to represent the flow or energy of life. It could refer to the life of an individual person or a family, or the life of an organization (Iwama 2006). In the metaphor of a river, the importance of context in shaping the river is emphasized. Rivers start because the moisture from rain and melting snow flows toward the lowest point of the land. Depending on the surrounding geography, rivers commence with varying amounts and types of water flow. They also flow toward lakes (some of which might be dry in lands such as Australia) and the sea. The course that the river takes depends on the unique combination of the surrounding geography, the strength of the river's water flow, and anything that lies in the river, such as rocks and driftwood. Similarly, the flow of the water can vary in different parts of the river as variations occur in the unique combination of the quality of the water flow and other elements of the river.

In the Kawa model, the river is used as a metaphor for the life journey, with birth being represented by the start of the river and end of life being the point at which the river flows into a larger body of water such as the sea. As Iwama (2006) explained, "An optimal state of

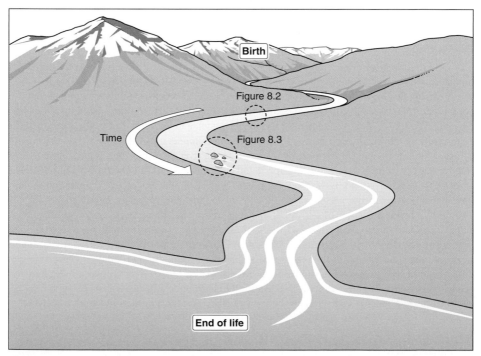

Fig. 8.1   The river. From Iwama MK. *The Kawa Model: Culturally Relevant Occupational Therapy*. Churchill Livingstone; 2006. Reproduced with permission from Elsevier Ltd.

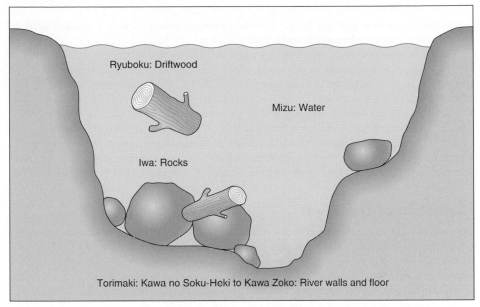

Fig. 8.2 Elements of the river. From Iwama MK. *The Kawa Model: Culturally Relevant Occupational Therapy*. Churchill Livingstone; 2006. Reproduced with permission from Elsevier Ltd.

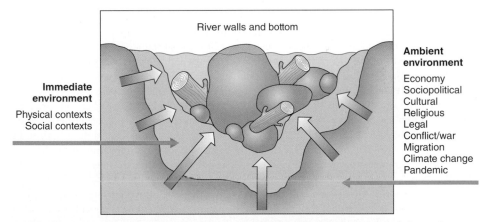

Fig. 8.3 Elements constricting water flow. From Iwama MK. *The Kawa Model: Culturally Relevant Occupational Therapy*. Churchill Livingstone; 2006. Reproduced with permission from Elsevier Ltd.

well-being in one's life or *river*, can be metaphorically portrayed by an image of strong, deep, unimpeded flow" (p. 143). As a metaphor for life, the river shows that people's lives are shaped by the unique contexts into which they are born and live as well as aspects of their own character and skill. Just as the river makes twists and turns, people's lives change in a variety of ways. Some of these changes can be anticipated, some are unexpected, some are shaped by the surrounding context, and some are primarily shaped by the flow of the water, which changes the shape of the river floor and walls. Sometimes the flow of people's lives is impeded by obstacles and at other times everything seems to flow easily. Some people are born into or live in circumstances that flow easily, like a wide river, and others' lives are characterized by obstacles that impact substantially upon their life flow.

While the river as a whole represents a person's life, a cross section taken at various points of the river would show different arrangements of the elements of the river. In certain places the river might be wide and deep, and the water flow might be largely unimpeded by obstacles. In other places it might be narrow and flow over rocks or drop in waterfalls. And in still other places the water flow might become impeded by debris or rock barriers that make the water stagnant. Similarly, the same section of river will look different at different times with varying rainfall, sometimes running strong and at other times essentially being a dry riverbed. In the Kawa model, attention is paid to both the river as a whole and to cross sections at different places. In the cross-sectional view, the various elements of the river are used as metaphors for different aspects of life.

Elements of the River

The first element in the Kawa model is water, or *mizu* in Japanese, which represents life energy or life flow. In many different cultures, water has symbolic meanings that relate to life. It is possible that water is a seemingly universal symbol of life because it is biologically essential for sustaining human life. Iwama (2006) highlighted that, while water is considered pure, cleansing, and renewing and is often associated with the spirit, culturally specific meanings for water also abound throughout the world. He encouraged people to explore what water symbolizes in the particular cultures with which they are engaging.

Water has a fluidity that allows it to flow over, around, and through a range of different obstacles and channels in its path. As a fluid it has the capacity to both shape and be shaped by whatever surrounds or contains it. It can take the shape of its container while also having the power to shape the objects and terrain it flows over or through. For example, the erosion that occurs in rocks that are exposed to water attests to its power to shape its surroundings. As Iwama (2006) stated, "Just as people's lives are bounded and shaped by their surroundings, people and circumstances, the water flowing as a river touches the rocks, walls and banks and all other elements of the river in a similar way to which the same elements affect the water's volume, shape and flow rate" (p. 144). He also explained how important this mutually influencing relationship between the water and its surroundings is to understanding collective cultures. He stated, "collectively oriented people tend to place enormous value on the *self* embedded in relationships. There is greater value in 'belonging' and 'interdependence', than in unilateral agency and in individual determinism. In such experience, the interdependent self is deeply influenced and even determined by the surrounding social context, at a given time and place, in a similar way to which water in a river, at any given point, will vary in form, flow direction rate, volume and clarity." (p. 145.)

Water also has the capacity to fill the spaces between other objects and only needs small spaces in which to flow. As a metaphor for life, this might suggest that life flow is possible in even the smallest of avenues. From the perspective of this metaphor, the task of an occupational therapist is to look at all aspects of the person's context of daily life and facilitate greater life flow. "When life energy or flow weakens, the occupational therapy client, whether defined as individual or collective, can be described as unwell, or in a state of disharmony" (Iwama 2006, p. 144). An occupational therapist can use any elements of the river, and their combinations, to work toward facilitating life flow.

Most recently, Iwama has begun to emphasize the importance of occupational therapists paying particular attention to the concept of spaces; to support and encourage the client to search for and identify the various channels of flow in their Kawa. Each channel or space between the hard structures (river walls and floor; rocks and driftwood) represents dimensions of the client's life that are still flowing, and perhaps more importantly, carry the potential and hope for greater flow.

Many Western occupational therapists have reported using and referring to the water and its various channels as occupation(s). By locating and naming the channels and spaces, opportunities, strengths, occupations, and "good points" of the client can be acknowledged, validated, and prioritized for the occupational therapy processes that will follow.

The next concepts are the *river walls and river floor*. In the Kawa model, the river walls and river floor are referred to as *kawa no soku-heki* and *kawa zoko*, respectively. Just as the walls and floor of the river shape its course, depth, and width, in the Kawa model these parts of the river refer to the contexts that surround clients; that is, their social and physical environments. Iwama (2006) emphasized that "these are perhaps the most important determinants of a person's life flow in a collectivist social context because of the primacy afforded to the environmental context in determining the experiences of self and subsequent meanings of personal action" (p. 146).

In this second edition, Iwama has expanded the river walls and floor by dividing them into two layers: proximal and distal. The *proximal layer*, which touches and directly shapes the water flow, remains the immediate social and physical environment. The new, deeper or distal layer acknowledges the presence and influence of ambient environmental factors that also contribute to the flow dynamics of the river. Socioeconomic status; political, economic, and religious conditions; and catastrophes such as wars and diaspora, earthquakes, pandemics, and climate change are some examples of distal environmental factors that can exert influence on the river's flow. The interrelations and interactions of these components determine the rate and quality of the water flow at each particular location and instance of the client's Kawa.

When discussing the river walls and floor, Iwama mainly attended to the social environment, thereby emphasizing the nature of a collectivist society to a Western audience. He stressed that the social environment chiefly refers to those people with whom clients have direct relationships and explained that the river walls and floor might represent family members, pets, friends, workmates, classmates, and so forth. He also emphasized that, in some cultures, the memories of departed family members can exert an important influence on people and that, in some cases, conversing with such departed relatives might constitute an important occupation for particular clients.

It is common for practitioners and clients situated in the Western world to interpret and use the Kawa model in a more individualist way. It is not unusual for these clients to emphasize or prioritize factors in the physical environment over those in the social environment.

When using the Kawa model and striving to gain a holist perspective, occupational therapists need to consider the various elements of the river together. Therefore, when thinking about the river walls and floor, it is important to understand that there is no particular shape that is "optimal." What matters is the amount of water that is able to flow through the placement, combination, and interaction of the various elements of the river. For instance, rivers that have reasonably narrow or shallow walls and floor might allow for adequate water flow if there are no obstacles blocking the flow. Similarly, a deep river that has been dammed will restrict the river flow in a way that is unrelated to the natural shape of the walls and floor. Metaphorically, the environment will certainly shape the life flow of a person's life, but this may be in a facilitatory or inhibitory way. Using the Kawa model, occupational therapists can look for ways to help shape the environment to facilitate the flow of the client's river and to enhance the harmony existing between clients and their contexts.

The third element of the Kawa model is *rocks*. The Japanese word *iwa*, which means large rocks or crags, is used in the Kawa model to represent life circumstances that are perceived by the client as problematic. Just as rocks can disturb the flow of water because of their shape, size, and placement in relation to the walls and floor of the river, rocks are used in the model to represent life circumstances that impede life flow. These life circumstances are considered by the client to be difficult to remove. The rocks in a person's life might be challenges that derive from bodily impairments that, in a particular environment, impede their life energy. Using the river image metaphorically, the flow of the water might be impeded when the unique size and placement of a rock forms a blockage in relation to the particular shape of the river walls and floor. However, in a river with differently shaped walls and floor, the same rock might have a minimal effect on the flow of the water. Thus it is important when using the model to discuss with clients the extent to which potential obstacles to life flow are perceived as actually impacting their lives.

Because each person's life circumstances and contexts are unique, the nature of the rocks and the blockages they form vary enormously. For some people, their rocks might relate to impairments of body structures and function; for example, symptoms and consequences of mental illness such as low motivation, anxiety, depression; and history of relapse; or nerve injuries; or medical conditions such as pulmonary emphysema. Other people might experience problems of performance such as difficulties with activities of daily living (ADLs) and self-care. Other rocks might include lack of money and human relations that are problematic, both of which illustrate that the obstacles in a person's life can arise from sources other than clients themselves.

The fourth element of the river discussed in the Kawa model is *driftwood*. The image of driftwood, *ryuboku* in Japanese, is used to represent:

personal attributes and resources, such as values (i.e., honesty, thrift), character (i.e., optimism, stubbornness), personality (i.e., reserved, outgoing), special skill (i.e., carpentry, public speaking), [and] immaterial (i.e., friends, siblings) and material (i.e., wealth, special equipment) assets and living situation[s] (rural and urban, shared accommodations, etc.) that can positively or negatively affect the subject's circumstance and life flow. (Iwama 2006, p. 149.)

Some of these examples of *personal attributes and resources* refer to features of an individual while others relate to that individual's immediate context and circumstance. While driftwood is also described as representing personal assets and liabilities, the concept of personal attributes and resources probably conjures a better image of what the driftwood is used to represent in the model. The image of assets and liabilities is often interpreted from an existential perspective to refer to characteristics that are within the person, whereas driftwood includes resources external to the person.

The utility of the concept of assets and liabilities lies in placing an emphasis on the fact that these attributes and resources can have a negative or positive effect on life flow. For example, Iwama (2006) provided a table listing examples of driftwood and, for each, positive and negative effects that each example might have on the life of an individual. Some of these are:

- Future expectations could have the positive effect of providing goals or something to look forward to, while potentially having negative effects by being a source of frustration, stress, and worry.
- The advantaged financial status of a child's parents could have the positive effect of assisting with equipment purchases and home renovations while also possibly facilitating increased dependency and contributing to a lack of skill development on the part of the child.

Compared with rocks, driftwood are a less permanent and more fluid feature of the river. Driftwood can be carried along with the water current and, depending on their shape and number, can become caught on rocks and combine to create a dam that restricts the flow of the water. Alternately, when carried by the strength of the water flow, they can also dislodge obstacles or carve channels in the river walls or floor, thereby increasing the flow of the water.

The final, but centrally important, element in the Kawa model is the *spaces* between obstructions. These are called *sukima* in Japanese and they help us understand the focus of occupational therapy from the perspective of this model. The elegant title of the section of his book in which spaces are discussed is "*Sukima* (space between obstructions) where life energy still flows: The promise of occupational therapy" (p. 151). In the Kawa model, the concept of *sukima* is based on an understanding of occupational therapy as a strengths-based approach. Rather than focusing on the remediation of problems, *sukima* emphasizes the importance of understanding where life is flowing in a client's situation and strategically working to maximize that flow.

While reduction in the size and shape of obstacles might be a strategy that can be used to maximize the life flow, it becomes only one of many ways to enhance life flow in those places in the river where it already exists. Focusing on the spaces *between* objects rather than the objects themselves, the Kawa model emphasizes the potential to facilitate life flow in a range of ways, including reducing the size and shape of problems, making channels in or changing the shape of the environment surrounding the client, and maximizing the power of the client's existing assets and resources. Using the metaphor of the river, the spaces where the water flows have the potential to increase because friction can wear away or dislodge those things that surround and impede the water's flow.

The River Metaphor

In conveying the relevance of the metaphor to occupational therapy practice, Iwama (2006) linked the concept of spaces to social roles and occupation. He explained by way of illustration that a functional impairment such as arthritis might be represented in the model by a rock, and the river walls might represent social groups or other people. The space between these two, through which the water flows, might represent a particular social role such as parent, worker, or friend which is successfully undertaken with arthritis. Iwama stated that "the spaces through which life flows, [are] representative of 'occupation', from an Eastern perspective" (p. 151). This linking of social roles and occupation is useful in understanding an Eastern comprehension of occupation. In collectivist societies, human action takes its meaning from the person's position in society. Therefore occupation becomes one vehicle through which individuals can fulfill their social roles. In other situations, for example, nonaction might be the way an individual can fulfill these roles.

Thinking about the river metaphor is useful in highlighting how the Kawa model is employed to understand a person's life flow and the role occupational therapy might have in facilitating this. The society in which people live shapes the kinds of roles they have (i.e., shapes the form and direction of the river), and obstacles that might relate to them and their circumstances (rocks) can impede their life flow and their ability to fulfill those social roles. Aspects of their character, skills, and circumstances (driftwood) are carried along by the water and may be able to flow through the river unimpeded or might become caught in the spaces between the river walls and floor and any rocks. Where driftwood contributes to a blockage of the river, it might impede the flow of water, or its damming effect might combine with the force of the water to dislodge obstacles or divert the water flow through new channels in the river walls and floor.

The fact that the water is frequently able to find new channels through which to flow provides the "promise of occupational therapy" (Iwama 2006, p. 151). It only takes a small space through which the water can flow to provide the potential for enhancing that life flow. Occupational therapists can use their creativity to work with clients or groups, and those connected to and instrumental in shaping clients' social roles, to seek ways to increase the channels through which the water can flow. Using the Kawa model, occupational therapists are encouraged to view each cross section of the river in a holistic way and keep in mind that the flow of water can be facilitated in a range of ways. Working to expand the current spaces through which water flows could be approached by exploring whether there are any ways that the walls and floor of the river could be shaped to increase this space, whether rocks could be moved or reduced in size, and how driftwood could best be used to enlarge the spaces that currently exist. The occupational therapist could also look for places where new channels of water could easily be opened (e.g., new social roles that might be available). Thus the river metaphor emphasizes that it is the unique combinations of and relations among the various elements of the river that form the basis for understanding a client's or group's current needs and the possibilities for addressing these needs within that particular circumstance. Box 8.1 presents a case illustration in which Kathy is working with a young man, Peter, and using the Kawa model to take a strengths-based approach to build on the spaces in which life is flowing for him.

BOX 8.1 ■ Case Illustration

Peter is an 18-year-old man who was referred to occupational therapy by a neurologist to support him in organizing his daily routine. He had been diagnosed with attention-deficit/hyperactivity disorder (ADHD) at the age of 12. He was in his first year of university at the time of the referral and had just completed his first semester. Unfortunately, he achieved a poor academic result because he forgot his weekly schedules, missed relevant information about assessments, and found it difficult to contribute to group assignments. Kathy, his occupational therapist, prepared for their first clinical encounter by reading the referral and his clinical file and devising some strategies that might help him organize his routine. She planned to use the Kawa model to guide her reasoning when gathering information and planning intervention.

In their session Kathy explained to Peter each element of the Kawa model and provided him with a diagram with each element and its meaning. As they talked and Peter drew, he would take his time, often thinking for long periods before drawing something. Kathy thought Peter looked sad while he was thinking and drawing. Peter's narrative started by describing a big flow of water cascading easily down the mountain but was soon blocked by a big rock. The rock represented the passing of his mother when he was 11 years old. She had been diagnosed with cancer. He was devastated because he really loved his mother and missed her greatly. She had been a very nurturing primary school teacher and the children in her class every year really looked up to her, as did he!

After that, the river walls and floor closed in around the big rock and many smaller rocks and driftwood were caught, obstructing the flow of the water. He identified that one of the pieces of driftwood that limited the flow was his difficulty expressing his emotions. This meant that he couldn't talk about his mother and his grief. There were many years where, each time he thought about his mother, he felt sad and tried to distract himself from his feelings by moving around the classroom, playing, and talking to his classmates. Teachers found this very disruptive and labeled him a troublemaker. Peter felt he was not understood by his teachers, the health professionals who assessed him, or the people in his family and community. Everyone seemed to take a punitive approach to his behavioral difficulties. And worst of all, because he was not doing well at school, he felt he could never follow in his mother's footsteps and achieve his dream of becoming a teacher.

On top of everything, the last couple of years of his primary schooling were affected by the COVID-19 pandemic. Because of school closures he had to stay at home and learn online. Kathy expected that Peter would have drawn an even more restricted river, because so many children and their families had found school closures so difficult. But Peter's river wasn't like this. Instead, the river walls were wider and there was more room for the water to flow. During this time, his father had been his main support. The wider river walls were because his father had created a positive environment that allowed Peter to learn. Together they had carved out spaces in the wall of Peter's river, and his life flow was less restricted. His self-esteem had improved, and he had experienced a sense of competence. In his drawing, the driftwood, his personal characteristics, had knocked away some of the small rocks. He felt he could finish high school and purue a teaching degree at university. By the time he went back to school, he seemed a very different person, more focused on learning and not disruptive in class, and he started to do well.

Now that he was at university, the river walls had closed in again, because there was less structure to scaffold his learning. He needed to develop new skills to cope with new demands. Through the Kawa model drawing and discussion, Kathy had gained a greater understanding of Peter's life and was able to identify aspects of it that made him feel happy, competent, and supported. She could see he had responded well to the supportive environment initially provided by his father and then by the high school. However, she knew the university environment required a greater level of organization and she planned to build on his strengths by helping him develop skills in time management, maintaining schedules, recording assessment due dates, and contributing to group work in a meaningful and timely way. She would combine working directly with him on skill development with connecting him to the learning support team at the university. Peter agreed to a referral to a psychologist to support his mental health. By using the strength-based approach inherent in the Kawa model, Kathy was able to work with Peter to enhance his potential and boost hope for greater life flow.

Historical Description of the Model's Development

The Kawa model was originally developed by a group of Japanese occupational therapists as a model relevant to Japanese culture, characterized by collectivism and hierarchy. As occupational therapy is a profession that developed in Western countries, the Japanese occupational therapists found that many of the assumptions upon which the theoretical basis of the profession was founded differed from their own understanding of life and the nature of humans. Iwama (2006) explained the problem that faced Japanese occupational therapists in trying to use concepts developed in Western countries within the context of Japanese culture. He stated:

> By trying to fit theory and assessments based on cultural patterns so remarkably different from those of the Japanese, a professional crisis was evident. The concepts of imported occupational therapy and theories have been left largely unreconciled to indigenous experience of reality. They are written in a foreign symbolic system (language) with many concepts having no direct equivalent in the Japanese lexicon. Their definitions are reduced to straight translations that are rote memorized, having the form of occupational therapy in the West but lacking meaning and the power to inform and guide a meaningful, valued practice. (p. 117.)

Although such cross-cultural dilemmas are made explicit in Iwama's work, he posited that similar cross-cultural challenges exist wherever the cultural norms that underpin the culture of Western occupational therapy, as embodied in its contemporary models, fail to resonate with the cultures of clients and with occupational therapists.

Iwama (2006) illustrated the problem of cultural translation of Western theory into Japanese culture through an anecdote about running a workshop for Japanese occupational therapists on occupational theory. He found that, at the end of the workshop, the participants did not understand the theories any better than when they had started. He gradually became aware that this workshop was probably one of many that the participants had attended in an earnest attempt to understand occupational theory. Japanese occupational therapists' pervasive experiences of difficulty understanding the theoretical concepts underpinning occupational therapy made Iwama think that the problem might lie in the cultural relevance of the theory, rather than in problems within participants. As he stated:

> Having no tangible narratives or models that held meaning within their own cultural understandings, Japanese therapists were reporting a certain degree of frustration regarding the lack of philosophical and ideological guidelines that defined occupational therapy in a comprehensible way. Their identities as occupational therapists were being jeopardized as they lacked meaningful theory that would aid them in explaining the scope and boundaries of their practice. (p. 119.)

This awareness provided the impetus for the development of a culturally relevant occupational therapy theory. Believing that, as occupational therapy had existed in Japan for 35 years, there must be some sort of tacit conceptual basis to the "forms of practice that were observable on the surface" (p. 120), Iwama approached a group of Japanese practitioners and made the suggestion (which he claimed "seemed audacious at the time" [p. 119]) that they develop their own model. This process resulted in the development of the Kawa model.

Japanese Cultural Context

Iwama (2006) claimed that three concepts fundamental to Western understandings of occupational therapy were critically challenged in the development of the Kawa model. These were "the central incumbency of the individual, a tacit understanding of humans as occupational beings,

[and] occupation typified as the interface between self and environment" (p. 139). Each assumption is discussed in the sections that follow.

CENTRALITY OF THE INDIVIDUAL

First, like many other Asian cultures, Japan is a collectivist culture in which the concept of a self that is separate from surrounding phenomena such as other people, plants, animals, and inanimate structures like rocks is completely foreign. In explaining the difference between this assumption and the Western worldview that shapes much of occupational therapy's perspective, Iwama (2006) described a Western view as an "existential perspective" (p. 142) in which the individual self is the focal point. This existential perspective is evident in terms such as *person-centered* and *client-centered* (where client is conceptualized as an individual). These terms are commonly used in occupational therapy discourse to emphasize the value placed on people, as distinct from bodies— hence contrasting a holistic perspective with a biomedical one. However, they also attest to the focus on individuals that is paramount in Western cultures.

In contrast, collectivist cultures view each individual as just one of many different elements that combine in a mutually influencing way to constitute life. The collective is the focal point of this cultural view and harmony within the collective becomes the goal, compared to individual mastery of the environment in an individualist culture. Iwama used the term *decentralized self* to refer to this concept of the self as "embedded in groups and inseparable from nature and environment" (p. 39). Iwama (2006) explained that the decentralized concept of self derives from the "East Asian cosmological myth or worldview, which configures the universe and all of its elements (including deities, natural flora and fauna, animate and inanimate matter) in one inseparable whole" (p. 41).

OCCUPATIONAL BEINGS

The second assumption challenged by Iwama is the concept of humans as occupational beings, which is central to much occupational therapy discourse. In relation to this premise, Iwama raises two issues for consideration. The first is whether humans are "occupational" by nature. The second deals with the doing, being, and becoming framework proposed by Wilcock (1998) that flows from the assumption that humans are occupational beings.

Regarding the assertion that humans are occupational by nature, occupational science concluded from empirical research that humans had a biological need for occupation. This assumption underpins the notion that engagement in occupation enhances health and well-being; that is, people need to do things to maintain their health and well-being. This assumption has been a core principle in occupational therapy theory since its foundation. For example, a well-known quote is that "man [sic], through the use of his hands as they are energized by mind and will, can influence the state of his own health" (Reilly 1962).

However, Iwama (2006) proposed that the concept of humans as occupational beings is based on an existential rather than collectivist understanding of humans and therefore might not have relevance for collectivist cultures. He explained that, from an existential perspective, humans obtain mastery over the environment by acting upon it. They exercise their personal agency. That is, through engagement in occupation they can be agents of change in the environment. The concept of mastery of the environment has been a central concept in occupational therapy theory since the early days of the profession. (The theory of Occupational Adaptation in Chapter 3 exemplifies the concept of mastery of the environment as a human need and refers to the work of Mary Reilly.)

This type of association between personal agency and action and health and well-being does not have relevance from a collectivist perspective, in that personal agency does not logically lead to enhanced health and well-being through mastery of the environment. As Iwama explained, "In the Japanese collective experience, more than the self, the group in which one holds membership is agent" (p. 51). In a collectivist society, persons and the environment are not juxtaposed and understood as separate entities but are all parts of the collective whole. Therefore, to enhance the health of the whole, individuals need to act *within* environments rather than *on* them. As the context within which one lives is part of the self, it makes little sense to attempt to maintain mastery over something that is, by definition, a part of one's self. Instead, health and well-being are associated with creating and maintaining harmony between people and the contexts in which they live. As Iwama (2006) explained, "states of well-being are contingent on human and natural relations... harmony between self and others and between selves and nature, forms the cornerstones on which 'security', belonging and states of well-being among Japanese people ultimately rests. The necessity to belong and the persistent drive for harmony form the basis to Japanese 'collectivism'." (p. 116.) Thus wellness is the result of harmony and balance between all elements in a person's life.

Emerging from the assumption that humans are occupational beings is the Doing, Being and Becoming framework. In this framework, Wilcock (1998) proposed that "*doing* well, well-*being* and *becoming* what people are best fitted to become is essential to health" (p. 255). However, Iwama (2006) demonstrated the culturally specific nature of this framework by articulating its lack of relevance to Japanese culture. He proposed that, to be more appropriate to Japanese culture, the order of the concepts should be *belonging*, *being*, and *doing* (rather than commencing with *doing* and then moving to *being* and *becoming*) because Japanese people are primarily accountable to their social relationships. As he stated, "matters of identity and meaning are ascribed in collective rather than in introspective processes . . . Roles are bestowed by the group and received by the individual, for no individual is considered greater than the collective. And once the role is made explicit, the self emerges to carry out the mandate of the collective." (p. 52.) Thus, in a collectivist society, belonging precedes and directs doing.

RECONCEPTUALIZING OCCUPATION

The third assumption critiqued by the Kawa model is that occupation is typified as the interface between self and the environment. As the first two assumptions have demonstrated, an existential approach assumes that the person and environment are separate, and that occupation provides the vehicle through which people can act upon the environment to master it. (The concept of mastery of the environment was evident in the occupational behavior approach of Mary Reilly and remains a central concept on the theory of Occupational Adaptation.) However, when moving away from this perspective, occupation and its purpose require reconceptualizing. From a collectivist perspective, individual action flows from one's place in the group and is a consequence of belonging, and the means through which one self actualizes. One's sense of self is developed by knowing and experiencing one's place within the context of the group and individual action gains its meaning in the context of the group. Therefore individual action is determined by the needs of the collective and engaged in by the individual because of their place within the group. Thus occupation is not a way of mastering the environment but a *consequence* of one's place in the group.

This difference has important implications for a conceptualization of occupation. In occupational therapy discourse, occupation has been defined as action that is meaningful to the person. In an existential culture, human action becomes meaningful to the individual when it relates to individual goals, interests, and values. In a collectivist culture, human action becomes meaningful to the individual when it serves the function of fulfilling the requirements of the collective and sustains the individual's position within the group. As Iwama (2006) stated, "In Japanese society, *doing* is important but may not mean much when separated from the social context in which it occurs and from which meaning is derived" (p. 116). Therefore the contextualized meanings of occupations have to be understood.

The difference in these perspectives is highlighted when considering the assessment and goal-setting tools used in occupational therapy practice. Because of the association made between (meaningful) occupation and individual goal setting, eliciting and establishing client-centered goals is the primary way priorities are set within client-centered occupational therapy practice. However, to determine meaningful occupation within a collectivist culture, assessments probably need to commence with an understanding of belonging rather than goals. Such an understanding would then allow the occupational therapist to work with the client to determine what kind of occupation could be used to support the client's sense of belonging.

Another aspect of Japanese society that differs from Western cultures is a different orientation to time. In general, Western cultures are future oriented. This is evident in occupational therapy practice through the emphasis on goal setting when aiming to be client centered. The assumption is that mastery of the environment is achieved by achieving goals. However, Japanese society is characterized by a temporal orientation that is located in the present. The implication for occupational therapy practice is that, rather than using therapeutic activity or occupations to meet goals (for the future), the process of therapy itself becomes most important.

Development of the Model

The Kawa model was developed by occupational therapists, educators, and students in Western Japan using a naturalistic research methodology that combined heuristic research and (modified) Grounded Theory. They used these qualitative research methods to "mine original concepts germane to their experience and interpretation of Japanese occupational therapy" (Iwama 2006, p. 120). They aimed to develop a conceptual model that was "derived from Japanese subjects, in Japanese language, using Japanese concepts and metaphors having high contextual meaning" (p. 120). Iwama claimed the Kawa model was one of the first of its kind in Asia where the tendency has been to import their theory from the Western world.

A group of 20 participants, representing a diversity of clinical practice backgrounds, met monthly in focus groups for approximately 6 hours per session over a 21/2-year period. In total, the group met over 50 times. The only inclusion criteria for these groups were that participants "had an interest in occupational therapy theory and desired to participate in making their clinical practice theoretically clearer" (p. 121). While grounded theory, which is widely used in Japan, provided the overall structure for the research, culturally relevant modifications were made to the process of collecting data. For example, as the social behavior of people in Japanese society is influenced by their place within the social hierarchy, they are likely to defer to the opinions of senior members of the group. To minimize such hierarchical influences on the data that were collected, three modifications were made: (1) making expectations clear that senior members of the group would both allow and encourage junior members to express their opinions, (2) using smaller subgroups to enhance the expression of a range of group members, and (3) using a range of data collection methods such as writing responses on cards and collectively developing drawn diagrams that did not rely on verbal expression in the context of the larger group.

A number of questions were used to generate data. Initially, two open-ended questions were used to focus the discussion: "How do you as Japanese occupational therapists conceive of the concepts of health and disability and illness?" and "What, if there is any, role or relation does occupational therapy have with these concepts?" These questions were used to explore the participants' perspectives of the meaning of occupational therapy in Japan. These questions were deemed important, as the identity crisis that occupational therapists appeared to feel was observed to be widespread. Subsequently, the general line of inquiry explored the question, "What is the meaning of Japanese occupational therapy?" Other questions were used to guide the inquiry more specifically and provide more structure for those who required it to complete the task. These included: "What is your role in Japanese society?"; "What do you do (in regard to intervention) and why?"; "Who are your clients?"; "What are you concerned with in your work?";

"How do you (Japanese OTs) define and regard 'health', 'disability'?" (pp. 126–127.) Data were recorded in the form of photographs of the sorted and assembled data, notes taken by participants were logged as data, and some sessions were videotaped.

Iwama (2006) described in detail the standard Grounded Theory process of analyzing the data inductively by coding the data using the early steps of open coding and axial coding, whereby data are "fractured" (p. 127) into minute sections and then combined into groupings of connected categories, respectively. Iwama remarked that, when explaining the codes produced in the axial coding stage, the participants explained each code in terms of its situational context. He suggested that "situational relativism was apparent throughout the procedure and highlighted the importance that context or 'ba' plays an important factor in the interpretation and judgment of realities for these Japanese therapists" (p. 127). Iwama (2006) also commented on participants' preference, when asked about the meaning of occupational therapy, to emphasize "life" and "life force."

Through the processes of grouping the data, five tentative thematic categories were developed (Iwama 2006, p. 128):

- Life flow and health
- Environmental factors (social, "ba," physical barriers)
- Life circumstances and problems
- Personal assets and liabilities
- Occupational therapy intervention

The final phase of data analysis in Grounded Theory is selective coding. In undertaking this process, in which a "central concept" is selected and related to the other categories, it became clear that no concept could be identified as more central than the others. Instead, all the concepts were linked and considered to be mutually influencing. As Iwama (2006) explained, "This configuration and structure could be described as a dynamic rubric in which a disruption or change in magnitude and quality of any one concept would affect the magnitude and quality of all of the other concepts." (p. 129.) He also described how, prior to the selective coding phase of data analysis, one participant's proposal that these five concepts and their interrelatedness could be better explained through the use of a river metaphor had been met with resounding acceptance by the whole group. This unanimous consent led to the use of the river metaphor, which appeared to be more consistent with a society "whose cosmologies are based on a naturalistic paradigm and whose ideations of humans are constructively inseparable from nature, society and deities" (p. 129) than a diagram consisting of boxes with arrows to show their relationships.

The river metaphor clearly resonated with the Japanese participants during the development of the conceptual model because it had specific cultural meanings. Iwama provided a quote from one of the Japanese research leaders in which she explained the central and symbolic place the river has in Japanese society and culture. After saying that, given the rich meaning of rivers in Japanese culture, it would seem superfluous to state that rivers are metaphors for life, she wrote:

> The river evokes in itself a very rich picture of mental imagery for a Japanese. A projection method developed in Japan called "fukei kousei hou" also uses the river as "a metaphor of unconscious flow". By looking at this holistic picture of our clients and by using such images that flow right deep inside our hearts, we may sympathize with their komari (problems) as people who live just like ourselves, otherwise we may understand their komari as something that happens to someone else somewhere in life. The clients that we treat and support are living persons. An approach without such sympathy carries the risk of being superficial and an affront to our clients. (p. 141.)

In this quote, she emphasized not only the rich cultural meaning of rivers in Japan but also that this kind of metaphor would help occupational therapists understand problems as human problems that touch us all.

Iwama (2006) emphasized that using the image of water flowing in a river to represent life flow also refocuses occupational therapy on facilitating life flow rather than increasing an individual's self-efficacy. In explaining the relationship between life flow and the important concept of occupation, Iwama stated:

> Occupation is reconceptualised to be the flow of water in this river. Without water flowing, there can be no river. Without occupation, in the context of this cosmological view of all elements in a frame or context inextricably connected, there can be no life. In this way, one's own or one's group's occupations are interwoven and connected to the occupation of others. Well-being is a collective phenomenon. Occupational therapy's purpose in this metaphorical representation of human being, then, is to enable and enhance life flow – a flow that encompasses self and context. (p. 144.)

Use of the Model in Practice

One of the ways the Kawa model appears to differ from many other occupational therapy models is its use in practice. The majority of occupational therapy models have been developed as theoretical perspectives that are used to guide occupational therapists in their conceptualization of humans and human occupation and performance and their consequent collection, organization, and integration of information. As such, the primary role of conceptual models is to guide and shape the perspectives of occupational therapists. This is an important function as it assists the profession to define its scope and focus and to articulate the uniqueness of its perspective on phenomena such as health and well-being. As a consequence, these conceptual models assist individual occupational therapists to confidently define the scope and focus of their practice in their local practice context and articulate their particular perspective. However, it is conceivable that the conceptual models that were developed were never intended to be shared with clients or other professionals. Instead, their value lies in providing an organizing structure to guide the practice of occupational therapists and a foundation from which they can use their interpersonal and professional skills to work with clients and professionals.

In contrast, the Kawa model was designed to be used as a basis for discussion with clients. In explaining this approach and with reference to a more traditional approach to theory, Iwama stated, "We may claim to be enacting client-centred practice, yet the clients' narratives are ultimately reduced, organized and made sense of through the structure, language and explanatory principles of our professional models and theories" (p. 159). In using the Kawa model, the client narrative is preserved as a whole and used as a basis for discussion.

In discussing using the Kawa model in practice, Iwama (2006) stated:

> There is not one "right" way to use and apply the Kawa model. The Kawa is a metaphor for life. The right way is realized when the model is adapted and used as a vehicle to illuminate the client's narrative for his or her life at a certain place and point in time. The Kawa model's ultimate form will be determined by the unique qualities of the client and the occupational therapy frame. (pp. 162–163.)

In emphasizing that there is no right way to use the model, Iwama also stressed that the metaphor of a river might not be the most appropriate metaphor to use for a particular client and an alternative metaphor can be used. The two principles that guide its use are that it honor the client (and their cultural context) and that the occupational therapist trust "that the client's narrative will emerge through a process of enabling him or her to do so" (p. 160).

While originally designed in the context of Japanese society, the Kawa model has been presented as a model that should be used and changed as appropriate to other cultural and situational contexts. As the only current occupational therapy model to address collectivist cultures, it represents a departure from traditional ways of thinking about human occupation and is likely to provide the catalyst for further development of other models appropriate to collectivist cultures.

Recent reports (Iwama 2009) on the applicability of the Kawa model suggest the model carries promise for use in individualist cultures as well.

The process of using the Kawa model in practice revolves around the drawing of a river (or other) diagram (or another form of creation of an appropriate metaphor). In doing this, the first decision should be about who will draw the diagram. Sometimes this might be the client and at other times it might be the occupational therapist in discussion with the client. In many cases the client is not limited to the individual but may consist of family members and/or others who represent the client's best interests. This is particularly seen in contexts of occupational therapy with children, people with dementia, persons with intellectual challenges, those with various mental health conditions, and so on.

In summary, the Kawa model was developed by a group of Japanese occupational therapists to develop an occupational therapy model that was culturally appropriate for them. Therefore the model does not purport to be relevant in its original form to all cultures. Instead, occupational therapists are encouraged to use metaphors (either of the river or something else if that works better) that have cultural significance to the people with whom they are working. In presenting the Kawa model, Iwama (2006) explained the cultural context it aimed to address. It is important that, in developing an understanding of the model, people understand the many cultural concepts that underpin it, such as the decentralized self within a collectivist culture. Unlike many other occupational therapy models, practitioners are encouraged to adapt the model for use in their local context.

Memory Aid

See Box 8.2.

BOX 8.2 ■ Kawa Model Memory Aid

Creation of the Client's River

Who (a person or collective) or what (organization, community, professional teams, etc.) is the client? How will the client's narrative be created? Will it be a river diagram? Who will draw it? In what context will it be discussed? How will I elicit the client's own words and perspectives and their descriptions of their circumstances?

Elements of the River

How are the elements of the client's river depicted at the moment?
- River walls and floor
- Rocks
- Driftwood
- Water flow (Where is this flowing at the moment? What is the river's history? How has the river been organized at different times?)

Significance of the Elements

What is the importance (relative size and shape) and meaning of each element of the river to the client? How do they affect the flow of the water? (in the present and past)

Change in the River

What could be changed (if anything could or needs to be) to increase the flow in the river?
If something changed in the river, how would this affect other elements?
What aspects of the river need to stay the same?
What would the occupational therapy contribution be to this change?
How would we know if the changes in the river were useful ones for the client?

Major Works

Iwama M. The Kawa Model: Culturally Relevant Occupational Therapy. Churchill Livingstone; 2006.

Conclusion

The Kawa model was developed by a group of Japanese occupational therapists because of the difficulty they were having understanding many of the occupational therapy concepts they were "importing" from Western countries. Therefore the focus of this model of practice is culturally relevant occupational therapy.

The model uses the metaphor of a river to represent life flow. The various elements of the river are used to represent different aspects of life in the context of a particular society. The river metaphor was chosen as it had particular meaning to Japanese people. Throughout the major text, Iwama emphasized the need to use the model in a way that is culturally relevant for both occupational therapists and their clients. Therefore the metaphor of a river should only be used if it has cultural relevance; otherwise, different metaphors should be selected.

In discussing the model, Iwama explained the nature of Japanese society, with its hierarchical structure and collective nature. Iwama also critiqued many accepted occupational therapy concepts relating to the nature of humans and occupation and explained how embedded they were in Western views of the world. For example, the primacy of belonging over doing in Japanese culture was explained. In these discussions, important cultural concepts were presented such as the decentralized self, the East Asian cosmological myth, and a Japanese cultural understanding of the world. Despite its purported benefits to practical application, the Kawa model's most important contribution to the discourse on theory in occupational therapy may be in its subtle influence on how power is structured and enacted in occupational therapeutic relationships. The Kawa model aims to privilege the unique narratives of each client, allowing the client to ultimately name the concepts and explain the principles that connect them. Whereas the conventional pattern of model use is for the theorist or therapist to create the concepts and principles of a model and apply them universally to all clients, the Kawa model aims to reverse this familiar power dynamic and make the client's unique story of their day-to-day realities the center of occupational therapy's concern.

The Kawa model is the only model of practice presented in this book that explicitly deals with collectivist cultures. People's social roles and relationships are at the center of their motivation for occupation. The purpose of the river metaphor is to facilitate discussion that leads to an understanding of the client's unique circumstances and needs. Unlike many other models, the Kawa model was devised to be used with clients. Its application to and use in a variety of cultures appear to have been rapid and broad, and readers are referred to the substantial literature and research that has been undertaken.

References

Iwama MK. The Kawa Model: Culturally Relevant Occupational Therapy. Churchill Livingstone; 2006.
Iwama MK, Thomson NA, Macdonald RM. The Kawa model; the power of culturally responsive occupational therapy. Disabil Rehabil. 2009;31(14):1125–1135. doi:10.1080/09638280902773711
Reilly M. Occupational therapy can be one of the great ideas of 20th century medicine. Am J Occup Ther. 1962 Jan-Feb;16 (1):1–9.
Wilcock A. Reflections on doing, being and becoming. Can J Occup Ther. 1998;65(5):248–257.

Reflections on Occupational Therapy Concepts

CHAPTER CONTENTS

Using Models in Practice   174

Trends in Occupational Therapy Theory   175
A Renaissance of Occupation   175

Conclusion   177

References   177

This chapter discusses how models of practice illustrate the trends in concepts and priorities in occupational therapy over time. Occupational therapy is a profession that exists within the broader context of societies. Consequently, the roles and perspectives of occupational therapy will differ from country to country, from place to place, and at different historical times. The models of practice presented in this book largely reflect the perspectives of occupational therapy in Western countries.

The only model included in this book that originated from a non-Western country is the Kawa model (Iwama 2006). In the first edition of this text, we explained that such models not only offer a novel and different perspective on occupational therapy but, because they emerge from a different worldview, they can help illuminate the cultural features of contemporary occupational therapy thought, theory, and practices. Such models can reveal the cultural situatedness of the profession's core concepts as well as the perspectives through which occupation is interpreted. We suggested that they highlighted how occupational therapy makes sense of and privileges the individual as the central concern through which occupations are interpreted, understands the relationship between individuals and environments, and conceptualizes occupation. We propose that awareness of and reflection upon these revelations can bring to debate how power is constructed and exercised in occupational therapy and is inherent in its values and procedures. In the first edition, we stated, "It will be interesting to see how this relatively recent acknowledgement of the Western-centric nature of occupational therapy theory plays out in the future." Now, a decade later, we are able to address the issue of how things *did* change in the intervening decade. Later in this chapter, we discuss trends in occupational therapy theory by commenting on the trends that were evident in the first edition of this book and reflecting on some emerging trends that are evident in the current versions of occupational therapy models.

This book presented a historical approach to models of practice. This approach provides a sense of the purposes for which they were developed, as well as situating them in historical time and place. Typically, models were developed to fulfill a perceived need in a particular context. In response, a model of practice was developed that identified limitations in the accepted views at the time and proposed alternative or extended perspectives. Local needs were often the impetus for the development of some of the other models covered in this book. In many cases, specific models were created to guide the development and implementation of a specific occupational therapy curriculum. In these cases, particular staff undertook the role of developing the model and they often then remained responsible for its further development. Other models were developed on behalf of national occupational therapy bodies. We explore three models reviewed in this book in terms of the issues they aimed to address when first developed.

The first example is the Model of Human Occupation (MOHO) (Kielhofner 1985, 1995, 2002, 2008; Taylor 2017). The first edition of MOHO was produced because of the perceived need to provide a structure that made explicit the relationships between the multitude of concepts generated within the occupational behavior tradition. Occupational behavior was developed by Mary Reilly at the University of Southern California in response to the limitations of a biomedical model of health and occupational therapy's alignment with it. The biomedical model of health was presented as mechanistic and reductionist in approach, characteristic of medicine and dominating health in the 1950s, '60s, and '70s, and at odds with occupational therapy values. Because this critique of a mechanical view of persons was central to both occupational behavior and MOHO, it is not surprising that the limitations of a mechanistic view of humans (upon which biomedicine is based) remained a theme throughout all editions of MOHO.

A second example is the Kawa model (Iwama 2006). This was developed because of the perception that a Western-centric understanding pervaded occupational therapy theory and the difficulty occupational therapists in Japan had in understanding many occupational therapy concepts because of poor cultural relevance. It also aimed to fill a gap in understanding diversity of cultural perspectives such as collective cultures, revealing occupational therapy's inherent Western-centric, individualist perspective. Because of its cultural emphasis and critique of Western-centric occupational therapy concepts, the Kawa model has had a broader appeal, resonating in countries other than Japan. The Kawa model was presented as a model that should be adapted as required to the cultural context in which it was being used, thus emphasizing the importance of cultural relevance.

A third example is the Canadian Model of Occupational Participation (CanMOP; Egan and Restall 2022). The models developed by the Canadian Association of Occupational Therapy (CAOT) demonstrate very clearly changing notions of the core concern of occupational therapy in the context of distinct historical times. The Canadian occupational performance model was used at a time when promotion of occupational performance was seen to depend on analysis and remediation of problems in occupational performance components. Subsequently, during the ecological turn in occupational therapy theory, the occupational performance model was replaced by the Canadian Model of Occupational Performance (CMOP). This new model enshrined the concept of client centeredness and presented the person, with a core of spirituality, surrounded by the environment. Important notions of occupational performance components—physical, affective, and cognitive—and performance areas—self-care, leisure, and productivity—were retained from the earlier occupational performance model. When the CMOP was revised, it was expanded from a focus on occupational performance to include the concept of engagement and became the CMOP-E. It also acknowledged the individualist assumptions inherent in occupational therapy; expanded the notion of client to include individuals, families, groups, communities, organizations, and populations; and recognized that clients had access to opportunities and included the notion of occupational justice. Finally, the CanMOP was developed in the historical time of the Truth and Reconciliation Commission of Canada (TRC) that was established to educate people about the history and legacy of the residential schools system. Consequently, the CanMOP is founded on acknowledgment of the effects of Canada's colonial past on people in the present day. It emphasizes the importance of occupational therapists working at micro, meso, and macro levels of context to address structural barriers to occupational participation.

Using Models in Practice

In this book, we presented models of practice as resources that can be used in and should *serve* practice. We aimed to present each model in an objective way, describing both the current version and placing it (and any previous versions) within a historical context. The purpose of doing this is to provide practitioners with a resource to use to support and enhance their practice. The specific situation in which an occupational therapist is located will shape their need for and use of models of practice. By reviewing brief overviews of each model, and comparing them, we anticipate that practitioners will be in a strong position to evaluate the potential utility of each model in their specific practice context. By understanding the main features of the model as well as the context within which it was developed and the gap or purpose it aimed to fill, practitioners are advised to make comparisons with the demands of their own roles, the needs of their own clients, and the nature of their organizational and social contexts. These comparisons can then inform their choices about which model(s) to use and how. We aimed to make the process of comparison easier by approaching each model in a similar way (main concepts and definitions of terms, and a historical description of the model's development) and providing a single-page memory aid. We also included case studies to illustrate some of the features of various models.

In addition to providing an overview of a range of different occupational therapy models, we also presented the Model of Context-specific Professional Reasoning (MCPR), a model for understanding how occupational therapists reason within specific contexts and how their thinking and action are intertwined. This model alerts occupational therapists to the complexity of contextual factors that influence their reasoning and decision-making, whether they are aware of it or not. The various different models also help shape their thinking, perceiving, and acting, depending on the demands of the roles practitioners are fulfilling. For example, if they are working directly with individual clients with a particular type of need, they might choose a model that helps them understand that need (possibly by providing the right amount of detail). Their role might involve designing programs for groups of people or they might be providing training to direct service providers. In such cases, other models might provide more support for them in that role.

As well as evaluating the potential utility of each model of practice to a particular practice setting, occupational therapists also need to consider how well each model resonates with their own professional reasoning styles. By that we mean that some models will align better than others with the ways a particular occupational therapist understands occupational therapy and the aspects of occupational therapy that they might particularly emphasize. For example, someone who emphasizes the role of the environment in their understanding of occupation is likely to find one of the ecological models most useful, someone who is more interested in understanding how the body works is likely to find one of the occupational performance models of greatest use, and someone who is especially concerned with social equity might find the CanMOP of particular use.

Professionals can use models of practice like a lens through which to create meaning in practice. Practice is complex and rarely presents in an organized or patterned way. Instead, it is the professional's job to make meaning and order from what can appear, at times, to be a chaotic mess. It is their job to organize information into meaningful patterns and clusters. Each model provides a lens through which to see practice. As with all lenses, they shape what people see and don't see, they guide them in their interpretation of what they see, and they magnify some aspects of the situation more than others. The vision they occupational therapists develop with the assistance of models can inform what action they will consider taking in aiming to better understand their client's situation and to provide a meaningful service.

Trends in Occupational Therapy Theory
A RENAISSANCE OF OCCUPATION

A major trend that occurred in occupational therapy theory was affirmation of the centrality of occupation. Kielhofner (2009) stated that occupation had served as a unifying concept in occupational therapy following the mechanistic period, during which the profession lost its identity as a unified whole. Whiteford et al. (2000) noted that occupational therapy had undergone a renaissance of occupation, in that it was returning to its founding roots.

However, the concept of occupation in occupational therapy has changed over time. The term was used during the founding period of the profession to refer to occupying time and having meaningful things to do. During the mechanistic period, occupation was approached in a very technical way in that it was primarily used as a tool to achieve specific goals. During that time, it was generally understood as a therapeutic means to an end and specific occupations were prescribed to achieve specific, normative goals. The models and their versions in the 1990s primarily emphasized occupational performance in context. While the *performance* of occupation remained the primary consideration, use of occupation in a direct cause–effect way was replaced with an ecological perspective on occupation. A person's occupational performance was understood to result from the interaction between the person and their environment.

The next phase encapsulated a broader understanding of occupation beyond occupational performance. Concepts such as participation in everyday life (Person-Environment-Occupation-Performance model or PEOP) and occupational engagement (CMOP-E) were added to the lexicon. To illustrate why occupational performance was too narrow to encapsulate the core concern of occupational therapy, Townsend and Polatajko (2007) provided a narrative about a severely disabled young man participating in marathons and triathlons with his father without "performing" these occupations. This broader understanding built upon the perception of people-in-context underpinning occupation as well as increased awareness that the notion of independence and the importance of individual action were Western assumptions and were not necessarily relevant to or valued in other cultures.

At the time of publication of the first edition of this book, the return to/renaissance of occupation was well embedded in current occupational therapy thinking. The link between occupation and social/occupational roles was also very much emphasized. The meaning and purpose of occupation was acknowledged as integral to people's participation in the society in which they live. There was also increasing acknowledgment that the structure of the society in which a person lives may advantage or disadvantage that person and that many people in their societies have unequal access to health services and resources. Consequently, occupational therapists' roles were increasingly seen as working with groups and populations, rather than just individuals, and might include activities other than direct service, such as policy development and advocacy.

The models presented in this second edition represent a further leap in the way occupation is conceptualized. We have referred to this current direction as a *transactional turn* in occupational therapy. A key characteristic of this phase is placement of occupation at the center, replacing the notion of client centeredness. For example, when discussing Collaborative Relationship-Focused Occupational Therapy with the CanMOP, Restall and Egan (2022) explained that client centeredness, which had been a core concept in CAOT publications since 1982, was a Western/Global North concept based on individualism. Instead, the CanMOP centers on occupational participation rather than on the person. Similarly, the Transactional Model of Occupation, upon which the OTIPM is based, has occupation at its center and conceptualizes occupation as the *result* of the transaction among seven contextual elements, one of which is the client. To occupational performance and participation, it also adds occupational experience.

The transactional turn in occupational therapy and the concept of occupation being the result of transactions is consistent with a Japanese collectivist understanding of occupation. Iwama (2003) explained that, in collectivist societies, people first belong and then act (i.e., their doing flows from their belonging). They are a part of the environment, and their place within that environment shapes and provides the impetus for action. Referring to the river metaphor, people act (occupation) according to the constellation of factors that make up the river at the time. Their action is shaped by and cannot be separated from the social and physical contexts in which they live.

Conclusion

Eleven occupational therapy models of practice were reviewed in this book. Taking a historical approach to these models highlights some of the trends and changes in occupational therapy theory and practice since the early 1980s. Readers are encouraged to refer to other texts for a more complete history of the profession and its ideas and for detailed descriptions of each model of practice. To this end, a list of the major publications has been included for each model of practice.

This review of the major models of occupational therapy practice since that time shows a trend away from the biomedical perspective that influenced health substantially from the 1960s, through an emphasis on a more biopsychosocial approach in the 1990s, toward a renewed focus on occupation from the end of the 20th century. Within this period of centering on occupation, there has also been a move from a focus on occupational performance to broader concepts of occupation that include occupational participation, experience, and justice. There has also been a move away from person centeredness to occupation centeredness. As models of practice embed the important theoretical concepts of occupational therapy, they provide a good way to understand the primary focus of occupational therapy at different times.

Models of practice are also developed to assist occupational therapists in putting theory into practice. In this book we have presented the models as tools that should serve practice. As professional practice requires decision-making and action under conditions of uncertainty, readers are encouraged to consider both their own ways of reasoning and the practice context within which they are reasoning and acting when making decisions about the potential use of models in their practice.

References

Egan M, Restall G. The Canadian model of occupational participation. In: Egan M, Restall G, eds. Promoting Occupational Participation: Collaborative Relationship Focused Occupational Therapy. CAOT; 2022:73–95.

Iwama M. The issue is...toward culturally relevant epistemologies in occupational therapy. Am J Occup Ther. 2003;57(5):217–223.

Iwama M. The Kawa Model: Culturally Relevant Occupational Therapy. Churchill Livingstone; 2006.

Kielhofner G, ed. A Model of Human Occupation: Theory and Application. Williams & Wilkins; 1985.

Kielhofner G. A Model of Human Occupation: Theory and Application. 2nd ed. Williams & Wilkins; 1995.

Kielhofner G. A Model of Human Occupation: Theory and Application. 3rd ed. Lippincott Williams & Wilkins; 2002.

Kielhofner G. A Model of Human Occupation: Theory and Application. 4th ed. Lippincott Williams & Wilkins; 2008.

Kielhofner G. Conceptual Foundations of Occupational Therapy Practice. 4th ed. F.A. Davis; 2009.

Restall G, Egan M. Collaborative relationship focused occupational therapy. In: M Egan M, Restall G, eds. Promoting Occupational Participation: Collaborative Relationship Focused Occupational Therapy. CAOT; 2022:97–117.

Taylor RR. Kielhofner's Model of Human Occupation: Theory and Application. 5th ed. Wolters Kluwer; 2017.

Townsend EA, Polatajko HJ, eds. Enabling Occupation II: Advancing an Occupational Therapy Vision for Health, Well-Being, and Justice Through Occupation. 2007 CAOT Publications ACE; 2007.

Whiteford G, Townsend E, Hocking C. Reflections on a renaissance of occupation. Can J Occup Ther. 2000;67(1):324–336.

INDEX

Note: Page numbers followed by *b* indicate boxes; *f* figures; *t* tables.

A

Accountability, 19–20
Acquisitional model, 106–107
Action
  art, science and, 28–29
  occupational therapy reasoning and, 34
  reasoned, 13, 22, 29, 34
  reasoning in, 29
Action domains
  adjustments and refinements, 149
  Canadian Occupational Therapy Inter-
    Relational Practice Process Framework,
    148–149
  co-design priorities, 149
  connect, 149
  explore occupational participation, 149
  plan for transition, 149–150
  seek understanding and define purpose, 149
Activities
  enabling, 44
  Occupational Performance Model
    (OPM), 41, 44
  see also specific types of activities
Activities of daily living (ADL), 41
Activity analysis, 92
Adaptation energy, 60–61
Adaptation gestalt, 59
Adjunctive methods, Occupational Performance
  Model (OPM), 44
Allen's Cognitive Levels Frame, 17
American Journal of Occupational Therapy, 130–131
American Occupational Therapy Association
  (AOTA), 40–41, 45–46, 87
Analysis of occupational performance,
  Occupational Therapy Practice
  Framework (OTPF), 93–94
Applied natural science, 13
Aristotle, 13–14
Art and science, 15, 28–29
Assessment
  Model of Human Occupation (MOHO),
    127–130, 127t
  Person-Environment-Occupation-Performance
    (PEOP) model, 81–82
Assets and liabilities, personal, 162
Autonomy, 137–138
  of professionals, 23
Axial coding, 169

B

Basic beliefs, 16
Behaviors, Model of Human Occupation
  (MOHO), 132–133
Biomechanical and Rehabilitative Frames, 17
Biomechanical model, 45
Biomedicine, 28
Blind spots, 20
Body element, Occupational Performance Model
  (Australia) (OPM(A)), 54

C

Canadian Association of Occupational Therapy
  (CAOT), 174
Canadian Journal of Occupational Therapy, 71
Canadian Model of Occupational Participation
  (CanMOP), 136–156
  case illustration, 151b
  client centeredness, 152
  collective level, 138
  components of, 137, 137f
  context, 139
  Critical Theory, 154
  definitions, 136–145
  Disability Creation Process (DCP) *vs.*, 154
  essential enhancements, 152
  historical description of development, 150–154
  individual level, 138
  International Classification of Function (ICF)
    vs., 154
  major concepts, 136–142
  meaning and purpose, 137
  memory aid, 154, 155b
  notion of history, 138
  occupational participation, 136–137, 139, 141,
    142–143
  occupational possibilities, 139
  occupational therapists, 143
  reasons for development, 174
  relationships and history, 138
  social determinants of health and health
    inequalities, 140–141b
  Social Model of Disability, 154
  transactional turn in, 176
  violence, 144
Canadian Model of Occupational Performance
  (CMOP), 18
  reasons for development, 174

Canadian Model of Occupational Performance and Engagement (CMOP-E) engagement aspect, 176

Canadian Occupational Therapy Inter-Relational Practice Process (COTIPP) Framework, 136, 146–150
  action domains, 148–149
  components, 150t
  connect, 149
  context, 146–147
  definitions, 146–150
  foundation process, 146
  major concepts, 146–150
  occupational consciousness, 147–148
  occupational participation, 146
  reasoning in, 148
  reflect, 147
  reflection on action, 147

Centrality of the individual, 166

Client centeredness, Person-Environment-Occupation-Performance (PEOP) model, 79

Client elements, 101

Client factors, occupational therapy domain, 91

Clients, definition of, 29–30

Clinical reasoning, 12, 26–27, 127.
  see also Professional reasoning

Codes of ethics, 24

Cognitive Behavioral Frames, 17

Cognitive capacity, Occupational Performance Model (Australia) (OPM(A)), 54

Cognitive context, 55

Collaboration, Person-Environment-Occupation-Performance (PEOP) model, 78

Collaborative Relationship Focused Occupational Therapy
  transactional turn in, 176
  trauma, 144
  values, 145

Collaborative Relationship-Focused Occupational Therapy, 136, 145
  contextually relevant relationships, 142–143
  definitions, 142–145
  major concepts, 142–145
  nuanced relationships, 143–144
  safety in therapeutic relationships, 144
  self-knowledge, 145

Collective level, Canadian Model of Occupational Participation (CanMOP), 138

Collectivist perspective, 157, 166

Common sense, 18

Communities
  influence of, 32
  of practice, 25–26

Compensation, Occupational Performance (OP) model, 42

Compensatory model, 106–107

Conceptual models of practice, 36

Conditional reasoning, 27

Connect, Canadian Occupational Therapy Inter-Relational Practice Process Framework, 149

Construct 1, Occupational Performance Model (Australia) (OPM(A)), 49–50

Context
  Canadian Model of Occupational Participation (CanMOP), 139
  Canadian Occupational Therapy Inter-Relational Practice Process Framework, 146–147
  Ecology of Human Performance (EHP), 73
  macro, 139
  meso, 139
  micro, 139

Contextually relevant relationships, 142–143

Control parameter, Model of Human Occupation (MOHO), 133

Critical Theory, Canadian Model of Occupational Participation (CanMOP), 154

Cultural beliefs, 33–34

Cultural context, 55
  Kawa Model, 165–168

Cultural practices, 25–26, 33–34

D

Decentralized self, 166

Decision-making
  process, 22–23
  see also Clinical reasoning; Professional reasoning

Declarative knowledge, 14

Department of Occupational Therapy, University of Kansas, 76

Diagnostic categories in medicine, 16

Diagnostic reasoning, 27

Dimensions of doing, 124–125

Disability Creation Process (DCP) *vs.* Canadian Model of Occupational Participation (CanMOP), 154

Disadaptive, 61

Doing, Being and Becoming framework, 167

Doing, dimensions of, 124–125

Domain, occupational therapy, 88–91
  categories of, 89
  client factors, 91
  environmental factors, 89
  performance skills, 90
  personal factors, 89

Domains, 16–17
  domain of concern, 16

Driftwood, Kawa model, 162

Dynamics systems theory, 132

E

Ecological models, 66–86. *see also specific models*
Ecology of Human Performance (EHP) model,
   17, 66, 73–78, 74f
   context, 73
   definitions of terms, 73–75
   environment, 73–74
   historical description of development, 76
   human performance, 75
   interventions, 75
   main concepts, 73–75
   memory aid, 77, 77b
   performance range, 74–75
   task, 74–75
Economic context, 55
Education and learning, 25
   sociocultural approaches to, 25
Education and teaching model, 106–107
Emergence, Model of Human Occupation
   (MOHO), 133
*Enabling Occupation: An Occupational Therapy
   Perspective,* 151–152
*Enabling Occupation II: An Occupational Therapy
   Perspective,* 152
Engagement *see* Canadian Model of Occupational
   Performance and Engagement (CMOP-E)
Environment, 166
   Ecology of Human Performance (EHP), 73–74
   Model of Human Occupation (MOHO),
      122–124
   Person-Environment-Occupation (PEO)
      model, 67
   social, 161
   see also Context
Environmental factors, occupational therapy
   domain, 89
Environmental impact, 123–124
Episteme, 13, 20
Epistemology, 13
Equipment
   Occupational Performance Model (OPM), 44
   use of, 44
Equity-based lenses, 148
Ethical code, 16
Ethical reasoning, 27
Evaluation
   Occupational Therapy Practice Framework
      (OTPF), 93
   Person Environment-Occupation-Performance
      (PEOP) model, 81–82
Evaluation and goal-setting phase, Occupational
   Therapy Intervention Process Model
   (OTIPM)
   finalize evaluation, 105–106
   gather initial information, 105

Evaluation and goal-setting phase,
   Occupational Therapy Intervention
   Process Model *(Continued)*
   global baseline, 105–106
   implement performance analyses, 105
Evidence-based practice (EBP), 15
Existential perspective, 157, 166
Expanded task analysis, 104
Expectations, 31–32
Experience, subjective, 120–121
Expertise, 23
   developing, 25. (*see also* Education and learning)

F

Felt space, 56
Felt time, 56
Fleming, Maureen Hayes, 27
Flexible structures, 53
Formal theory, 14
Foundation process, Canadian Occupational
   Therapy Inter-Relational Practice Process
   Framework, 146
Frames of reference, 16, 17
   overarching, 17
   see also Models; *specific models*
Functions, elements of, 41

G

Generalization reasoning, 28
Geopolitical elements, 101
Government processes, 33
Grounded Theory, 168
Guidelines for practice, 16

H

Habits
   definition of, 117–118
   of occupational performance, 118
   occupational therapy domain, 90
   of routine, 118
   of style, 118
   see also Habituation
Habituation, 113, 114, 117–120
Heterarchy, Model of Human Occupation
   (MOHO), 132, 133
Hierarchy, Model of Human Occupation
   (MOHO), 133
History, Canadian Model of Occupational
   Participation (CanMOP), 138
Homeostasis, 61
Human ecology, 67, 74f
Human occupation, 114. *see also* Model of Human
   Occupation (MOHO)
Human performance, Ecology of Human
   Performance (EHP) model, 75

Hypotheses, favored, 20
Hypothetico-deductive reasoning, 26–27

I

Individual centrality, 166
Individual level, Canadian Model
  of Occupational Participation
  (CanMOP), 138
Influences, 31
Interaction
  with people, 29–30
  Person-Environment-Occupation (PEO)
    model, 67–68
Interactive approach, Person-Environment-
  Occupation (PEO) model, 67
Interactive reasoning, 27
Interest, Model of Human Occupation (MOHO),
  116–117
Intergenerational trauma, 144
Internal context, Occupational Performance
  Model (Australia) (OPM(A)), 50–55
Internalized roles, 119
International Classification of Function (ICF)
  vs. Canadian Model of Occupational
    Participation (CanMOP), 154
Interpersonal capacity, Occupational Performance
  Model (Australia) (OPM(A)), 54
Interventions
  assessing outcomes of, 127
  Ecology of Human Performance (EHP)
    model, 75
  implementing, 127
  Occupational Performance Model
    (OPM), 42–45
  Occupational Therapy Practice Framework
    (OTPF), 93–94
Intrapersonal capacity, Occupational Performance
  Model (Australia) (OPM(A)), 54
Iwa, 161–162
Iwama, Michael, 157

J

Japanese cultural context of the Kawa
  model, 165–168
  centrality of the individual, 166
  occupational beings, 166–167
  reconceptualizing occupation, 167–168
Judgement, 24

K

Kawa model, 18, 157–172, 174
  case illustration, 164b
  definitions of terms, 157–160
  development of, 168–170
  elements of the river, 160–163

Kawa model (Continued)
  historical description of development, 165
  Japanese cultural context, 165–168
    centrality of the individual, 166
    occupational beings, 166–167
    reconceptualizing occupation, 167–168
  main concepts, 157–160
  memory aid, 171, 171b
  river metaphor, 157–160, 158f, 159f, 163
  use in practice, 170–171
Kawa no soku-heki, 161
Kawa no zoko, 161
Knowledge
  applied body of, 16
  declarative, 14
  different types of, 13–14
  fundamental body of, 16
  implications of different types of, 15
  nonpropositional, 14, 22
  personal, 15, 22
  procedural, 14, 22
  propositional (scientific), 14, 22
  theoretical, 16
  types of, 13–14, 22
  valuing of, 15
Knowledge base, 23

L

Legislation, 33
Legitimate tools, 16
Leisure occupations, 52–53
Lenses, Model of Context-specific Professional
  Reasoning (MCPR), 31–32
Life circumstances, problematic, 161–162
Life Course perspective, 138
Life energy/flow, Kawa model, 160
Lifespan perspective, Model of Human
  Occupation (MOHO), 125–126
Lived body, 120–122

M

Macro context, 139
Mastery, 166
Mattingly, Cheryl, 27
Mechanistic view, Occupational Performance
  Model (OPM), 46
Meso context, 139
Metaphors
  Kawa model, 157–158, 158f, 159f
  river, 157–160, 158f, 159f, 163, 176
  window, 125
Micro context, 139
Mind element, Occupational Performance Model
  (Australia) (OPM(A)), 54
Mixed-models approach, 106–107

Model of Context-specific Professional Reasoning (MCPR), 35b, 29–36, 30f, 175
  background features, 32–34
  diagrammatic representation, 30f
  foreground features, 31–32
Model of Human Occupation (MOHO), 18, 113–135
  assessment tools, 127–130, 127t
  case illustration, 130b
  definitions of terms, 113–124
  dimensions of doing, 124–125
  elements and components, 115t
  environment, 114, 122–124
  habituation, 113, 114, 117–120
  historical description of development, 130–133
  interest, 116–117
  lifespan, narrative approach to, 125–126
  lived body, 120–122
  main concepts, 113–124
  memory aid, 134b, 133
  pathways of change in, 126
  performance capacity, 114, 116, 120–122
  personal causation, 114–115
  personal convictions, 116
  reasons for development, 174
  sense of obligation, 116
  use in practice, 127–130
  values, 116
  volition, 113, 114–117
Models
  of practice, reasoned, 34–36
  terminology, 16–17
  using in practice, 174–175
  see also specific models
Motor capacity, Occupational Performance Model (Australia) (OPM(A)), 54
Motor control model, 45
Motor skills, 90, 124–125

N
Narrative reasoning, 27
Nonpropositional knowledge, 14

O
Objective components of performance, 120–121
Objects, 123
Occupation
  Occupational Performance Model (OPM), 45
  Person-Environment-Occupation (PEO) model, 69
  reconceptualizing, 167–168
Occupational Adaptation Model (OAM), 17, 39–65, 60f
  conceptual framework for, 61–62
  definitions of, 59–62

Occupational Adaptation Model *(Continued)*
  historical description of model's development, 62
  main concepts, 59–62
  memory aid, 63, 63b
  occupational response, 60–61
  role expectations, 59–60
Occupational analysis, 92
Occupational behavior, 17
Occupational beings, 166–167
Occupational consciousness, Canadian Occupational Therapy Inter-Relational Practice Process Framework, 147–148
Occupational experience, Transactional Model of Occupation, 100–101
Occupational forms, 124–125. *see also* Tasks
Occupational justice, 89–90
Occupational narratives, 125
Occupational participation, 124–125
  Canadian Model of Occupational Participation (CanMOP), 136–137, 139, 141, 142–143
  Canadian Occupational Therapy Inter-Relational Practice Process Framework, 146
Occupational performance
  definition, 41
  development of, 41
  habits of, 118
  Model of Human Occupation (MOHO), 124–125
  Person-Environment-Occupation (PEO) model, 70, 70f
  Person-Environment-Occupation-Performance (PEOP) model, 78
  Transactional Model of Occupation, 100–101
Occupational Performance Model (Australia) (OPM(A)), 39–40, 47–58, 49f
  construct 1, 49–50
  core elements, 54–55
  definitions of, 48–56
  external context of, 48, 55–56
  features of, 48–49
  historical description of model's development, 56–57
  internal context of, 48
  main concepts, 48–56
  occupational role, 50–52
  performance areas, 50–52
  performance capacities, 53–54
  performance units, 53
  person-context-performance relationship, 51
  space and time, 56
Occupational Performance Model (OPM), 39–65, 41f
  definitions of terms, 40–42
  historical description of model's development, 45–46

Occupational Performance Model *(Continued)*
  intervention, 42–45
  main concepts, 40–42
  memory aid, 58, 58b
  performance areas, 41
  performance components, 42, 43t
  performance contexts, 42
  see also specific models
Occupational possibilities, Canadian Model of
  Occupational Participation (CanMOP), 139
Occupational profile, Occupational Therapy
  Practice Framework (OTPF), 93
Occupational role
  definition, 41
  dimensions of, 52
  Occupational Performance Model (Australia)
    (OPM(A)), 50–52
Occupational therapists, Canadian Model of
  Occupational Participation (CanMOP), 143
Occupational therapy, domain of, 87
*Occupational Therapy Guidelines for Client-Centred
  Practice,* 150–151
Occupational Therapy Intervention Process Model
  (OTIPM), 87–112
  case illustration, 108b
  definitions of terms, 99–100
  evaluation and goal-setting phase, 105
  historical description of development, 108–109
  intervention phase, 106–107
  major concepts, 99–100
  memory aid, 110, 110b
  reevaluation phase, 107
  Transactional Model of Occupation, 100–102
  true top-down reasoning, 102–104
Occupational Therapy Performance Framework
  (OTPF), 40
  participation, 124–125
*Occupational Therapy: Performance, Participation,
  and Well-Being,* 78, 82
Occupational Therapy Practice Framework
  (OTPF), 17
Occupational Therapy Practice Framework:
  Domain and Process, 87
Occupational Therapy Practice Framework, fourth
  edition (OTPF-4), 87
  case illustration, 96b
  definitions of terms, 88
  domain, 88–91
  environmental factors, 89
  historical description of development, 96–97
  intervention, 93–94
  major concepts, 88
  memory aid, 97, 98b
  outcomes, 95
  process, 89
  professional reasoning, 92–93

*Occupational therapy: practice skills for physical
  dysfunction,* 40
Occupational therapy process, 91–96, 91f
  assessment/evaluation phase, 81–82
  intervention phase, 82
  Person-Environment-Occupation-Performance
    (PEOP) model, 80–82, 81f
Occupational Therapy Product Output Reporting
  System, 96–97
Occupational Therapy theory trends, 175–176
Occupation-based models, 17. *see also specific models*
Occupations
  defined, 69
  leisure/play, 52–53
  Occupational Therapy Practice Framework,
    fourth edition (OTPF-4), 88–89
  productivity/school, 52–53
  rest, 52
  self-maintenance, 52–53
Open coding, 169
Open systems theory, 132
Order out of Chaos, 132
Organizational context, 32–33
Overarching frames of reference, 17

P
Paradigms, 16–17
Participation, Transactional Model of Occupation,
  100–101
Patient
  definition in Occupational Performance Model
    (OPM), 40–41
  see also Clients
Patient-reported outcomes (PROs), 95
Pedretti, Lorraine Williams, 40
People, interaction with, 29–30
Performance, 176
  objective components, 120–121
  subjective components, 120–121
  see also Occupational performance
Performance areas
  Occupational Performance Model (Australia)
    (OPM(A)), 50–52
  Occupational Performance Model (OPM), 41
Performance capacity, 114, 116, 120–122
  Occupational Performance Model (Australia)
    (OPM(A)), 53–54
Performance components, Occupational
  Performance Model (OPM), 42, 43t
Performance contexts, Occupational Performance
  Model (OPM), 42
Performance patterns, occupational therapy
  domain, 90
Performance range, Ecology of Human
  Performance (EHP) model, 74–75
Performance skills, 90

Performance units, Occupational Performance Model (Australia) (OPM(A)), 53
Person
  Ecology of Human Performance (EHP), 74
  Person-Environment-Occupation (PEO) model, 67
Personal attributes and resources, 162
Personal causation, 114–115
Personal convictions, 116
Personal factors, occupational therapy domain, 89
Personal knowledge, 14, 22
Personal theory, 14
Person-Environment-Occupation model (PEOM), 66, 67–73, 68f, 74f
  advantages of, 71
  components, 67–68
  definitions of terms, 67–71
  historical description of development, 71–72
  main concepts, 67–71
  memory aid, 72, 72b
  occupational performance, 70, 70f
  transactive *vs.* interactive approach, 67
Person-Environment-Occupation-Performance (PEOP) model, 17, 66, 78–85, 79f
  client centeredness, 79
  components, 79
  definition of terms, 78–80
  historical description of development, 82–83
  main concepts, 78–80
  memory aid, 83, 84b
  occupational performance, 78
  occupational therapy process, 80–82, 81f
  performance aspect, 176
  systems perspective, 78–79
Perspectives, 16–17
Phenomenology, lived body, 120–122
Philosophical assumptions, 16
Philosophies, 16–17
Phronesis, 14, 20
Physical context, 55
Physical environment, 123
Physical environmental elements, 101
Physical space, 56
Physical time, 56
Plato, 13
Play occupations, 52–53
Play or leisure activities, 41
Plots, Model of Human Occupation (MOHO), 125
Political context, 55
Powerful Practice, 99
Practical wisdom, 13–14
Practice, 12–21
  communities of, 25–26

Practice *(Continued)*
  defining, 12
  gap between theory and, 15
  models serving, 18–19
  nature of professional, 23
  reasons for, 12
  scope of, 19
  terminology, 15–18
  using models in, 174–175
Pragmatic reasoning, 27
Pragmatism, 19
Procedural knowledge, 14, 22
Procedural reasoning, 27
Process
  occupational therapy, 91–96, 91f
    categories of, 91–96, 91f
  skills, 90, 124–125
Productivity occupations, 52–53
Professionalism, 19–20
Professional practice
  nature of, 23
  see also Practice
Professional reasoning, 19, 22–38
  art, science and action, 28–29
  background features, 32–34
  communities of practice, 25–26
  foreground features, 31–32
  historical view, 26–28
  model, 29–34, 30f. (*see also* Model of Context-specific Professional Reasoning (MCPR))
  nature of professional practice, 23
  occupational therapy, 26–28
    and models of practice, 35b, 34–36
    reasoning and action, 34
Propositional knowledge, 14, 22
Psychological context, 55
Purposeful activity, Occupational Performance Model (OPM), 44

Q
Qualitative research, 29
Quantitative research, 29

R
Reasoned action, 12, 22, 34
Reasoning
  in action, 29
  Canadian Occupational Therapy Inter-Relational Practice Process Framework, 148
  clinical *see* Clinical reasoning
  conditional, 27
  diagnostic, 27
  ethical, 27

Reasoning *(Continued)*
  generalization, 28
  interactive, 27
  narrative, 27
  pragmatic, 27
  procedural, 27
  professional *see* Professional reasoning
  scientific, 27
  therapeutic, 127, 128t
  true top-down, 102–104
  types of, 27
Recovery Model, Canadian Model of
    Occupational Participation (CanMOP), 154
Reflect, Canadian Occupational Therapy
    Inter-Relational Practice Process
    Framework, 147
Reflection-on-action, Canadian Occupational
    Therapy Inter-Relational Practice Process
    Framework, 147
Reilly, Mary, 131, 174
Relatedness, 137–138
Relationships
  Canadian Model of Occupational Participation
    (CanMOP), 138
  contextually relevant, 142–143
  nuanced, 143–144
  person-context-performance, 51
  person-environment, 67
  person–professional, 33
  professional, 26
  between professionals and clients, 33
Relative mastery, 61
Remediation, Occupational Performance Model
    (OPM), 42
Renaissance of occupation, 46, 175–176
Rest occupations, 52
Restorative model, 106–107
Rights-based lenses, 148
Rights-based self-determination, 144–145
River floor, Kawa model, 161
River metaphor, Kawa model, 157–160, 158f, 159f,
    163, 176
River walls, Kawa model, 161
Rocks, Kawa model, 161–162
Role expectations, Occupational Adaptation
    Model (OAM), 59–60
Roles
  internalized, 119
  occupational *see* Occupational roles
  occupational therapy domain, 90
  social, 25
Routines, 53
  habits of, 118
Routines, occupational therapy domain, 90

Rse justice-based lenses, 148
Ryuboku, 162

S
Safety in therapeutic relationships, 144
School occupations, 52–53
Science and art, 15, 28–29
Scientific knowledge, 14
Scientific reasoning, 27
Selective coding, 169
Self-determination, rights-based, 144–145
Self-knowledge, Collaborative Relationship-
    Focused Occupational Therapy, 145
Self-maintenance occupations, 52–53
Self-organization, 132–133
Self-regulation, 23
Sense of competence, 137–138
Sense of obligation, 116
Sensory capacity, Occupational Performance
    Model (Australia) (OPM(A)), 54
Sensory context, 55
Serving practice, models, 18–19
Skills
  communication, 124–125
  interaction, 124–125
    Model of Human Occupation (MOHO), 124–125
  motor, 124–125
  process, 124–125
Social context, 55
Social determinants of health and health
    inequalities, 140–141b
Social environment, 123, 161
Social environmental element, 101
Social interactions skills, 90
Social Model of Disability, Canadian Model of
    Occupational Participation (CanMOP), 154
Social roles, 25
Sociocultural elements, 101
Space and time, 56
Spaces
  Kawa model, 163
  Model of Human Occupation (MOHO), 123
Spirit element, Occupational Performance Model
    (Australia) (OPM(A)), 55
Spiritual context, 55
Style, habits of, 118
Subjective components of performance, 120–121
Subjective experience, 120–121
Subtasks, 53
Sukima, 162
Systems perspective, Person-Environment-Occupation-
    Performance (PEOP) model, 78–79
Systems theory, Model of Human Occupation
    (MOHO), 131

T

Tasks, 53
  Ecology of Human Performance (EHP), 74–75
  elements, 101
  Person-Environment-Occupation (PEO)
    model, 69
Teaching, 25
Techniques, 16–17
Temporal elements, 101
Terminology, 15–18
Theoretical foundations, 16
Theoretical knowledge, 16
Theory, 12–21
  application of to practice, 24
  defining, 12
  formal, 14
  gap between practice and, 15
  levels of, 18
  personal, 14
  reasons for, 12
  terminology, 15–18
Therapeutic reasoning, 127, 128t
Therapeutic relationships, safety in, 144
Therapeutic use of self, 92
Thoughtful action, 25
Three track mind, 27
Time, space and, 56
Traditional task analysis, 104
Transactional Model of Occupation, 99, 100–102
  occupational elements, 100–101
  occupational experience, 100–101
  occupational performance, 100–101
  situational elements, 101
  transactional turn in, 176
Transactive approach, Person-Environment-
  Occupation (PEO) model, 67

Transgenerational trauma, 144
Trauma, Collaborative Relationship-Focused
  Occupational Therapy, 144
Treatment approaches, 16–17
Trends in occupational therapy theory, 175–176
True top-down reasoning, 102–104
Trustworthiness, 23–24
Truth and reconciliation Commission of Canada
  (TRC), 174
Two-body practice, 15, 28

U

Uncommon sense, 18
*Uniform Terminology for Reporting Occupational
  Therapy Services*, 96–97
University of Kansas, Department of Occupational
  Therapy, 76
University of Southern California, 131

V

Values
  Collaborative Relationship-Focused
    Occupational Therapy, 145
  Model of Human Occupation (MOHO), 116
Valuing of knowledge, 15
Violence, Canadian Model of Occupational
  Participation (CanMOP), 144
Volition, 113, 114–117

W

Water, Kawa model, 160
Window metaphor, 125
Work and productive activities, 41
World Federation of Occupational Therapists
  (WFOT), 25
  website, 88–89